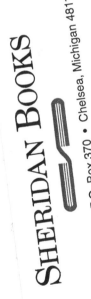

SHERIDAN BOOKS

140 Buchanan St. • P.O. Box 370 • Chelsea, Michigan 48118

Title: GEM/SCHULTHEISS/BODIES AND SOULS
Best Way Debbie Sayers

Job:145555-002 Smyth Case Bind

Acct # 290327
AE:12

HARVARD HISTORICAL STUDIES, 139

Published under the auspices
of the Department of History
from the income of the
Paul Revere Frothingham Bequest
Robert Louis Stroock Fund
Henry Warren Torrey Fund

Bodies and Souls

Politics and the Professionalization of Nursing in France, 1880–1922

Katrin Schultheiss

HARVARD UNIVERSITY PRESS

Cambridge, Massachusetts

London, England · 2001

To Eric

Library of Congress Cataloging-in-Publication Data

Schultheiss, Katrin.
Bodies and souls : politics and the professionalization of nursing
in France, 1880–1922 / Katrin Schultheiss.
p. cm. — (Harvard historical studies ; 139)
Includes index.
ISBN 0-674-00491-4 (alk. paper)
1. Nursing—France—History.   2. Nurses—France.
3. Professional socialization—France.   4. Nurse and physician—France.
I. Title.   II. Harvard historical studies ; v. 139.

RT12.F4 S4 2001
610.73′0944—dc21   00-061391

Acknowledgments

Many individuals and institutions on both sides of the Atlantic made possible the research for this book and the dissertation upon which it was based. I would like to acknowledge the generous financial support of the Franco-American Commission for Educational Exchange, the Krupp Foundation, the Sheldon Fellowship Foundation, and the Minda de Gunzburg Center for European Studies at Harvard University.

The archivists at the Municipal Archives of Lyons and Bordeaux and at the Archives of the Assistance Publique and the library of the Croix-Rouge Française in Paris, Jean Valette at the Departmental Archives of the Gironde, and Jacqueline Roubert at the Archives of the Hospices Civils of Lyons generously made available a wealth of material, both catalogued and uncatalogued, going out of their way to find any shred of documentation on nurses.

My sincerest thanks to my advisers at Harvard, Patrice Higonnet, Olwen Hufton, and Caroline Ford, who encouraged me to think about gender issues in French history and offered much helpful advice, criticism, and encouragement. Margaret Darrow provided thoughtful comments on this manuscript as well as on conference papers and articles composed over the years of our mutual research and writing on French nursing. Jo Burr Margadant and John A. Davis raised important interpretive questions about portions of this project. On the other side of the Atlantic, Mihaela Bacou and Danielle Haase-Dubosc at the Reid Hall Program, and Yvonne Cohen and Evelyne Diebolt helped make my stay in Paris both fruitful and enjoyable.

Though less easily quantifiable, the fellowship of good friends facilitated this project in crucial ways. Mary Kne, Janet Lindsley, Mindy Roseman,

Benjamin Schmidt, Scott Smith, and Jean Weiss provided intellectual, emotional, and spiritual support through many years of researching and writing.

My family has been a constant source of inspiration and sustenance. My mother, Ulla Schultheiss, a nurse herself, in many ways embodies the very combination of selfless devotion and professional expertise idealized by French reformers a century ago. I have no doubt that she served, however unconsciously, as the initial inspiration for this project. My father, Peter Schultheiss, through his dedication to intellectual inquiry and devotion to teaching, has served as an inspiration of an entirely different sort. I am grateful for their unwavering faith in me.

My children have also, despite themselves, spurred me on to finish this book. Rachel, Samuel, and William have collectively forced me to become more efficient and trained me to work well into the night. Their exuberance and joyousness, as well as their own trials and tribulations, always put the frustrations of academic work in perspective; their "contribution" continues to be immeasurable.

My deepest gratitude is reserved for Eric Arnesen, whose intellectual and emotional support has been indispensable throughout this long process. Eric read every word of this manuscript and the multiple versions that preceded it; his incisive comments have been invaluable. He voluntarily played the roles of unofficial research assistant, copy-editor, editor, and critic, always with characteristic enthusiasm and energy. But more importantly, his constant encouragement and belief in the importance of this project quite literally made it possible. I dedicate this book to Eric in gratitude, admiration, and with love.

Contents

Introduction

A large crowd gathered in the immense Salpêtrière Hospice on January 29, 1898, to honor the nurse Marguerite Bottard on the occasion of her appointment to the order of Knights of the Legion of Honor. One after another, representatives from the hospital administration and medical staff, from the city council and the national government, stepped to the podium to praise the devotion, selflessness, and virtue of this woman whose life of service stood as a model for all lay nurses. "Never has the Legion of Honor Cross been better placed than on your chest," declared Dr. Paul Raymond, for whom Bottard had worked for the past five years:

> Thus have fifty-seven years of loyal service been rewarded, service rendered in situations that are among the most difficult and delicate of those conferred upon women. This occupation requires absolute abnegation, unqualified devotion, and a love of one's fellow being that is rarely found, even among women, to the degree that it is found in you. You have done your duty, your entire duty, without fanfare, in a simple, I would say saintly, manner.[1]

Raymond's encomium signified more than simply reverential, if paternalistic, praise for a faithful subordinate. His choice of words—"absolute abnegation," "unqualified devotion," and especially "saintly" duty—invoked phrases commonly used to describe the Catholic nursing orders that still shaped public discourse about the hospital nurse. In the minds—or at least in the rhetoric—of those assembled, Bottard's service proved that nursing was not the exclusive province of nuns but belonged to all women. Her life and the official recognition accorded to it powerfully symbolized the potential of applying such inherently feminine talents as devotion, delicacy, and self-abnegation to public service. Bottard was celebrated as a model nurse precisely because she exhibited all the qualities of a mother without having a family; because she performed her work in a "saintly manner" out of "devotion" and "love of [her] fellow being" that carried not a trace of desire for personal fulfillment, ambition, or material gain.

The praise and official honors that were bestowed upon Bottard (she had already received the state-administered *palmes académiques,* bronze and gold medals from the Assistance Publique (AP) administration, and a special medal in recognition of fifty years of service) stood as public reminders of the state's humanitarian face. Bottard's portrait, one of the very few likenesses of actual nurses to be published in Paris in the prewar years, served as a perfect iconographic symbol for the new lay nurse. In the oft-reproduced etching, the aging woman's stern yet sympathetic gaze stares unflinchingly at the viewer. Her broad shoulders give her an almost soldierly, masculine appearance, and the tricolor ribbon of the Legion of Honor, the sanction of the state, is displayed like a military medal on her lapel. The imposing portrait, a study in strength and competence, was a fitting icon for the AP administration still struggling in 1906 to establish the legitimacy and the reputation of its lay nursing staff.

From a historian's perspective, Marguerite Bottard's story is noteworthy not only for its symbolic content but also because Bottard is one of only a few nurses from the prewar period whose life story has not vanished from the historical record. Indeed, by the time of her death in 1906, Bottard had become something of a celebrity among Paris Assistance Publique administrators, physicians, and employees. The seventy-six-year-old head nurse (*surveillante*) had spent more than half a century in the Salpêtrière Hospice for women, almost all of that time in charge of wards filled with epileptics, hysterics, and other victims of severe mental disorders. Bottard's eulogists never tired of relating her biography, a veritable parable of a life of feminine virtue. Born in 1822 to small farmers in the Cote-d'Or in Burgundy, Marguerite Bottard was the fourth of fifteen children. In 1841, after a series of bad harvests forced her parents to sell their land, she moved to Paris, where one of her older sisters worked as a servant to a low-level administrator at the Salpêtrière. Having decided that she would "prefer to serve the poor than the rich," Marguerite took a position as ward maid (*fille de service*) at the hospice. After six months she moved up several ranks to *suppléante,* where she remained for ten years. In 1852, she was appointed to the position of *sous-surveillante,* ministering to the mentally ill, and nine years later she became a *surveillante,* the highest post in the nursing hierarchy.[2]

Bottard rarely left the institution, and she was reputed to have stayed within its premises for six years at a stretch on several occasions. "A voluntary recluse," an obituary in the Paris journal *Le Progrès médical* noted with reverence, "she dedicated every moment to [her patients], all her life . . . forgetting herself completely in order to think only of her duty of affectionate devotion."[3] Marguerite Bottard represented the virtuous potential of every poor young woman, and the numerous official honors bestowed upon her affirmed the state's approbation of this particular type of female public servant.

But Bottard's fame did not stem from the length and quality of her service alone. It was her position as head nurse under one of the nation's most prominent medical practitioners, Jean-Martin Charcot, that ensured her celebrity status. Bottard's function in the eminent neurologist's service exceeded that of able assistant at his lectures and exemplary nurse to his patients. More than one colleague of Charcot's recalled her successful efforts to calm an agitated doctor or to mediate among fractious or jealous students.[4] As a nurse, Marguerite Bottard facilitated the genius of Charcot and the training of his disciples, her admirers implied. In so doing, she served as a model for what nursing might become in the age of medical progress. Secular nurses could and should retain the most important characteristics associated with religious nurses: dedication, humility, deference, and self-abnegation. To Charcot and many others at the forefront of modernizing medical care in France, the ideal nurse closely resembled a nun without a habit. Even in a republic explicitly dedicated to the principle of secularizing public life, efforts to laicize and modernize the public hospital nursing staffs were strictly limited by the ubiquitous association of female public service with religious vocation.

The transformation of the nursing profession during the four decades surrounding the turn of the century was shaped by the political and cultural tensions of the early Third Republic. Nursing evolved during this period from a vocation dominated by Catholic nursing orders assisted by untrained lay women and men and largely invisible to politicians, to a "feminine profession" that included increasing numbers of lay women yet continued to accommodate thousands of experienced religious women.[5] In the 1870s, the wards of almost all of France's 1,500 hospitals were run by about 11,000 members of active religious congregations. By the turn of the century that number had risen to about 12,000 and by 1911 to about 15,000. At the turn of the century, France had approximately 200 female religious orders providing nursing care. At the same time, lay hospital staff (not all of whom were nurses) grew from about 14,500 in 1880 to more than 20,000 in 1900 and almost 95,000 by 1911.[6]

The burgeoning number of lay personnel did not, however, signal a wholesale secularization of nursing; nor did it mark the establishment of a modern profession for women.[7] Government officials' efforts to secularize public institutions were often at odds with their own goal of improving the quality of nursing care in the country's antiquated hospitals. Anticlerical doctors and policymakers, hoping to drum up replacements for thousands of experienced religious nurses, quickly found their ambitions thwarted by strong cultural beliefs about the appropriate role of women in the new republican social order—beliefs often held by the anticlerical reformers themselves. One such reformer, the physician and politician Désiré Magloire Bourneville, led a thirty-year campaign to replace the *congréganistes* (religious sisters) employed by the Paris Assistance Publique administration with lay nurses. Recognizing that the existing lay staff was not yet prepared to step into the sisters' supervisory roles, Bourneville established the country's first public, part-time nurse-training programs, drawing on the working- and peasant-class nursing personnel already employed in the hospitals. He and his fellow reformers argued that these "women of the people" could earn a respectable living in the hospitals while securing the republic's control over its health-care institutions. Bourneville's efforts to eliminate religious nurses from the hospitals, though ultimately successful, met with resistance not only from the expected clerical sources but from doctors who argued that "womanhood," synonymous with motherhood, was incompatible with nursing. Only the "unsexed" religious sister who had replaced service to the family with service to God could devote herself to caring for the sick who were not her own.

The defenders of the religious nurses in Paris were no match for the hostile and powerful municipal council that controlled the hospitals' budgets. But in Lyons, where a financially autonomous hospital administration appointed by the prefect could afford to ignore the dictates of the city government, religious nursing prevailed. What is remarkable about the Lyons *hospitalières* is less that they survived well into the twentieth century; it is, rather, that they were held up as a model for nursing in the republic not only by Lyons' hospital administrators and clerical supporters but also by the city's powerful doctors' association and reformers in the national government. Although organized along congregational lines with religious habits and a regular prayer schedule, the *hospitalières* had no mother superior and answered only to the secular administration. All but the most extreme anticlerical republicans agreed with the *Petit Journal* of Paris that the Lyons sisters represented an "ingeniously practical and very felicitous 'concordat'" between lay authority and religious personnel.[8] The Lyons *hospitalières* retained all the desirable qualities of religious women—humility, self-abnegation, and obedience—while lacking the autonomy and power of a full-fledged religious order.

To the majority of republican reformers, the Lyons sisters were a far more suitable model for the "republican nurse" than that provided by the educated, highly trained career nurses who graduated from the new nursing schools of Bordeaux. Spearheaded by the Protestant doctor Anna Hamilton with support from the mayor, Dr. Paul-Louis Lande, the rigorous training programs aimed to turn nursing into a highly skilled profession for educated, middle-class single women. Hamilton and Lande, basing their reforms on the work of England's Florence Nightingale, believed that the modern nurse must be secular, female, single, well-educated, and trained not only in a classroom but in a functioning hospital ward. But like Nightingale, the Bordeaux reformers stressed the need for the nurse to recognize in herself a vocation to devote her life to bringing enlightened care to the sick and injured. As trained professionals, these women would take their place by the doctor's side as purveyors of uniquely feminine scientific expertise. To the Bordeaux reformers, being a woman was a necessary but not sufficient condition for becoming a nurse. Their initiatives quickly garnered accolades from abroad but met with resistance from doctors, who feared such nurses would threaten their recently established professional boundaries and their growing authority in the hospital. The professional nurses also encountered hostility from their own colleagues, the working-class men and women who constituted the majority of the hospitals' "secondary staff." The latter sought to claim nurses and other medical support staff for the ranks of the working class, and thus came in direct conflict with those reformers who viewed nurses as models for modern, independent women.

The beginning of the First World War marked a major turning point in the public image of the nursing profession. The influx of tens of thousands of middle- and upper-class volunteer nurses into wartime hospitals and aid stations recast the various conceptions of nursing into one of feminine patriotic service. Minimally trained but eager to make herself useful, the volunteer nurse of World War I appeared in the press, in novels, and on placards as a surrogate mother and sister, selflessly using her inherently feminine capacity for comfort and healing to minister to the fallen warriors of the nation. The wartime experience catapulted the reputation of nursing from an occupation still performed predominantly by poor peasant and working-class women or by members of religious congregations, to an admirable, indeed heroic, activity for all French women. But the praise accorded the wartime nurse was praise not for her skill and expertise but for her essential womanhood turned to patriotic purposes. Bordeaux's Anna Hamilton and other proponents of professional nursing repeatedly voiced their frustration, sometimes shading into despair, at the war-induced decline in training standards. Nursing had become a form of public motherhood.

In the immediate postwar period, new opportunities opened up for nurses. The human toll exacted by the war, including the millions killed and wounded and the millions more who fell victim to tuberculosis, influenza, and a host of fatal childhood diseases, accelerated the mounting panic over France's low birthrate. In hopes of staving off demographic catastrophe, the government enlisted hundreds of nurses and volunteer "visitors" to teach domestic hygiene and the methods of proper infant and child care. These women—both full-time trained professionals and part-time volunteers—entered the homes of the poor and the working class to evaluate their health, secure treatment where necessary, and instruct them in effective techniques for the prevention of tuberculosis and the promotion of children's well-being. Nursing in the postwar years was confirmed as a form of public, scientific motherhood. Indeed, it was as a form of public motherhood that nursing became firmly attached to the national project of rejuvenating and regenerating the exhausted population.

Finally, in 1922, the state established a national diploma for nursing along with a set of national guidelines for training. Though certainly a mark of legitimacy, the national nursing diploma had, perhaps not surprisingly, ambiguous significance for advocates of reform. The diploma was not required to practice nursing, and schools were not required to conform to the established standards. The 1922 legislation emerged from nursing leaders' desire to establish officially that nursing was a trained profession and not simply a gender attribute. The new regulations constituted the state's response to the demand for standards in a field that seemed to bear an increasingly weak relationship to concrete training and skills, and an increasingly strong relationship to womanly duty.

The irony of this dilemma for advocates of professional nursing was that they themselves, of course, had grounded their reform efforts in no small part in women's supposedly innate aptitude for nursing. Women's inherent maternal instinct and capacity for gentleness and sympathy suited them for very particular public roles and conformed neatly to prevailing gender norms. In the short run, the equation of essential femininity and professionalization served reformers well in gaining significant official and public support for the complete feminization of the profession. Advocates of religious and secular nursing alike could agree that nursing belonged, naturally, to women. But reformers also insisted that nursing required both a solid basic education and extensive professional training. Here they suddenly encountered resistance, again from across the political spectrum. As long as nursing was understood to be a natural attribute of womanhood, it could at once be considered useful and important, yet subordinate and unthreatening. Once reformers demanded rigorous training as well as substantive authority for nurses as medical professionals, politicians, administrators, and doctors alike balked. Many objectors urged continued support for religious nursing, which remained safely within the realm of charitable work and never really threatened the authority of the ascendant medical profession. Those whose politics could not accommodate the presence of congregations in public hospitals carefully limited the amount of training and the autonomy they were willing to grant to lay nurses.

It is important to remember that nursing reformers throughout Europe and the United States all faced the problem of promoting a skilled profession rooted in an essentialist identity. Nurses everywhere faced the additional challenge of establishing professional autonomy while affirming their subordinate position in the medical hierarchy. Yet by the early twentieth century, English and American nurses had successfully carved out a place for themselves as medical professionals. French lay nurses, in contrast, faced a much more ambiguous future. Religious nurses still ran the wards of many municipal institutions and still dominated popular imagery of nurses. Lay nursing was still widely associated with domestic service, charitable duty, noblesse oblige, and, briefly, feminine patriotism. In a society long accustomed to regarding women's work as mediated either by the Church or by the family, the notion of a female professional was at best an unfamiliar concept. Thus the models that won the most widespread acclaim at the national level were the Lyons *hospitalières*, who acted ostensibly from religious motivation but obeyed a secular authority, and the wartime volunteer nurses and visiting nurses of the postwar period, whose services and skills were understood to derive most directly from their essential feminine role as mothers. Those who, like Anna Hamilton, believed that the elevation of nursing from domestic service to professional status depended most crucially on its identity as a feminine occupation requiring years of specialized training and a middle-class moral code, found that in the early Third Republic "feminine profession" was as much an oxymoron as "female citizen."

The inability of reformers in France to effect nationwide changes in the recruitment, training, and practice of nursing had its immediate cause in disagreements within the ranks of the reformers about the goals they were trying to achieve. While some honestly wanted to improve the quality of nursing care, others sought above all to remove the religious nursing sisters from hospitals; while some viewed nursing as a working-class occupation and thus sought to improve salaries and working conditions, others hoped to turn it into a middle-class profession, the equivalent of teaching. More fundamentally, however, the difficulty of establishing uniform nursing standards and practices in France had its roots in the social and political issues that shaped the early Third Republic. The debate over nursing reform reflected widespread uncertainty over the future of women's role in the new republican social order, calling into question the relationship of women to work, and the relationship of women, in general, to Church, family, and, ultimately, the state.

The historical literature on the nursing profession has, with only a few exceptions, remained largely the province of nurses themselves. Within the academy, the history of nursing appears to have fallen between the cracks, with scholars interested in women's professions concentrating on teachers or, to a lesser extent, on civil servants, and those interested in women's work focusing on industrial and domestic production. Historians of medicine have traditionally accorded nurses a paragraph or two at best. At the same time, social historians of religion have tended to study the "contemplative orders" that bore the brunt of anticlerical wrath or the teaching orders, whose eviction from public schools became nearly synonymous with secularizing and "republicanizing" the minds of French children.

A few notable exceptions to this general oversight do exist. The eminent historian of medicine Jacques Léonard was the first to recognize the continuing significance of Catholic nursing orders throughout the nineteenth century, pointing out the deeply rooted historical connection between women religious and the healing arts.[9] Colin Jones built on this thesis by examining the controversies surrounding religious nursing in the eighteenth and early nineteenth centuries.[10] Véronique Leroux-Hugon's work on the development of lay nursing in Paris has brought to light a wealth of new material, but is necessarily limited by her focus on the always exceptional case of Paris. While the debate over anticlericalism affected nursing reform throughout the country, Paris stood alone in the speed and definitiveness with which it cast off its religious nursing staff.[11] Evelyne Diebolt's account of Anna Hamilton's work at the Maison de Santé Protestante in Bordeaux, written at the request of the institution itself, serves largely as a tribute to Hamilton's work and neglects to consider her efforts in the broader political context. The more comprehensive *Cornettes et blouses blanches,* edited by Yvonne Knibiehler, as well as Marie-Françoise Collière's *Promouvoir la vie* and Geneviève Charles's *L'Infirmière d'hier à aujourd'-hui,* provide more sweeping views of the development of modern nursing through the late twentieth century.[12] All are attentive to the dual roots of nursing in religious and maternal duty while presenting the landmark events in the modernization of the profession. As the first full-length historical works dedicated to nursing, these survey texts are certainly significant additions to the corpus of scholarship on women's professions. But the history of nursing can and should be examined with broader questions in mind.

My own research suggests that the very different experiences of nursing reformers in Paris, Lyons, and Bordeaux were the product of conflicting beliefs about woman's "natural calling," her status as an individual, her duty to the republic, and her place in public institutions. Local political, cultural, and economic circumstances often tipped the scales in favor of one or another definition of womanhood; none of them was self-evident and none predetermined by the establishment of the republic. This book, then, uses the transformation of the nursing profession in the decades before and after the turn of the twentieth century as a lens through which to examine the social, cultural, and political meanings of womanhood at a particularly crucial moment in the formation of the modern French republic.

Historians agree that efforts to define republicanism during this period centered in no small measure on establishing the inherent opposition between the secular, rational republic and the obscurantist, authoritarian reign of the Church. Indeed, anticlericalism and hostility to Catholicism served as a rallying cry for moderate and radical republicans from the 1870s until the passage of the law separating Church and state in 1905.[13] As the historian Ralph Gibson has observed, the conflict between Catholics and republicans frequently attained "the levels of bitterness of a religious war."[14] The importance of secularism to the definition of the republican political and social order can be seen most clearly in the government's sustained efforts to create secular public schools throughout the country. Only lay teachers could form young republican minds; only through secular schools could the state guarantee the future of the secular democratic political order.[15]

But if publicly educated children represented the future of the republic, women's recalcitrant religiosity indicated how far away the goal of a secularized society remained. Membership in female religious orders in France soared over the course of the century from 12,300 in 1808 to 135,000 (excluding Alsace and Lorraine) in 1878. Nearly 400 female religious orders were founded between 1800 and 1880, by which point 7 out of every 1,000 women belonged to a religious order, compared with about 4 out of 1,000 on the eve of the Revolution.[16] The Church, despite its insistence that women belonged in the home tending to their families, provided numerous opportunities for female employment. Beginning in the seventeenth century and continuing into the twentieth, religious orders involved with poor relief frequently established workshops where their impoverished clients would, purportedly, learn useful skills along with the discipline and moral rectitude that comes from hard work. By the middle of the nineteenth century, the largest such establishments were attached to convents that "employed" sometimes as many as 100,000 girls and single women in the silk and clothing industries.[17] At the same time, membership in an active religious congregation afforded single women of all classes the opportunity to perform a vast array of social services, including nursing and teaching. Although these service-oriented congregations were legally abolished during the Revolution, they were quickly reinstated under Napoleon and enjoyed unprecedented growth throughout much of the nineteenth century.

Officials of the early Third Republic routinely accused the Church of attempting to control women through confession and through coerced membership in religious congregations. As late as 1907, two years after the passage of the law separating Church and state, Georges Clemenceau warned the nation that "the number of [women] who escape the domination of the clergy is ridiculously low. If the right to vote were given to women tomorrow, France would immediately jump backwards into the middle ages."[18] Ideas about women's inherent emotional and sexual vulnerability served to promote images of a seditious, grasping clergy seeking to undermine the republic and male authority in the family by claiming the hearts, minds—and in some alleged incidents, the bodies—of its women.[19]

It comes as no surprise, then, to find the anticlerical city councils of both Paris and Lyons attempting to replace their religious nurses with secular staff. What is more intriguing, however, are the objections to secularization that were raised in both cities, objections that prevailed in Lyons but fell short in Paris. In both cities, anticlerical doctors, hospital administrators, and politicians—many of whom unequivocally supported the laicization of the nation's schools—rallied to the defense of the congregational nurses. Even the physicians in parliament hesitated to advocate secularization of the hospital nursing staffs. As historian Jack Ellis has noted, "Few could ignore the risks involved in attacking the very popular sisters, and few had any ideas as to who would replace them."[20] Even strong supporters of the laicization of the nursing corps admitted that there simply were not enough competent lay nurses to take the place of the *congréganistes* should they be evicted. In Ralph Gibson's words, the female congregations "found themselves in a crucial conjuncture where the demand for [their medical and social] services was expanding, and nobody else cared much to satisfy it."[21]

Pragmatic explanations for the staying power of the hospital sisters go a long way toward elucidating the apparent contradiction between the Third Republic's approach to the schools and its approach to the hospitals. Not only did the country lack professional training programs for nurses, but few lay women viewed hospital nursing as a career option. Long hours and low wages coupled with an unpleasant, hazardous work environment made it an unattractive alternative even to domestic work. The common requirement that the nursing staff remain in residence on the hospital premises—usually in cramped, unhygienic, uncomfortable dormitories—further reduced the appeal of nursing to all but the most economically desperate or the most selfless believers in charitable duty.

Yet practical considerations alone do not adequately explain why there was so little concern that the nurses in most of the nation's public hospitals were members of Catholic religious orders. After all, France prided itself on being at the forefront of scientific progress, and its parliament included unprecedented numbers of doctors who consistently pressed for public health legislation. Yet French hospital nurses were trained only through experience on the wards, and their very religion preached the subordination of the inherently corrupt body to the perfectible spirit. Pragmatism also does not explain why there was so little interest in establishing standardized professional training programs that would be the first step to building a corps of competent lay replacements for the religious sisters.[22] As the Bordeaux reformer Anna Hamilton never hesitated to point out, such programs had been functioning in England and the United States for decades. Pragmatic concerns cannot explain the fervor with which someone like surgeon Armand Desprès, a Protestant self-described anticlerical Freethinker, defended the religious nurses of Paris, nor why ninety doctors and surgeons would sign a petition formally protesting the laicization of the capital city's hospitals and hospices.[23] Even more tellingly, invocations of practical concerns cannot explain why the nursing sisters of Lyons not only survived repeated efforts to replace them, but were held up by republicans of all stripes as a national model for nursing in the new republic.

Republican support for religious nursing stemmed not only from pragmatic concerns but from more deeply rooted beliefs about women's role in the republic. Throughout the nineteenth century, French economists, social theorists, and public officials of all but the most radical left-wing political persuasions understood that the value of women's work derived from its direct relationship to the most important cultural and social institutions of the time: the Church and the family. Republicans, for all their emphasis on the inherent value of work, were no different. Formulations dating back to the Revolution endowed only men's labor with intrinsic worth; women's work received its meaning through the institutions it served. The family structured women's unpaid labor in the home and justified their performing wage labor to support their children, siblings, or parents. This rationalization of women's work became particularly important in the closing decades of the nineteenth century, when concern about *dénatalité*—the low national birthrate—and high infant-mortality rates led to scores of studies of the effects of employment on women's reproductive and maternal capacities. In addition, fears of social and political turmoil associated with increasing Socialist and trade unionist activity and the nascent women's rights movement made the family the focus of many republican quests for stability and national rejuvenation. Women's work could be justified only insofar as it helped strengthen the family.[24]

The revolutionary period's redefinition of work as a free and direct contract between citizens, and the concomitant elevation of work to the status of the fundamental right and obligation of all Frenchmen, were both profoundly gendered transformations.[25] The eighteenth-century revolutionaries who, in eradicating the guild system, declared the transparency of all relationships between men, by the same logic excluded women from citizenship on the grounds that all their interactions with society were necessarily mediated. The characterization of women's work as labor performed for an intermediary social grouping stood in stark contrast to ideas of men's work as both ennobling to the individual and essential to the state. The connection between men's work and the state was perceived as at once direct and abstract, whereas the connection between women's work and the state was obscured by its allegiance to other institutions and more concrete in its direct application to real social entities. The notion that women could, through their labor, contribute to the greater social good directly and as individuals, without such mediation, was deeply problematic even to the staunchest opponents of religious congregations. Older notions of women's work died hard, even in the context of rapidly advancing medical science and fervent anticlericalism. Many republicans—physicians included—remained resistant to a concept of nursing that rejected the corporate form of organizing women workers, advocated the acquisition of sophisticated expertise (both strategies implying an acceptance of professional individualism), and denied the primacy of the family in the hierarchy of women's social obligations.

While the role of gender in shaping the anticlerical discourse of the period has long been noted, the relationship between gender ideology and late-nineteenth-century French republicanism has only more recently received attention. Steven Hause and Anne Kenney pioneered this theme, arguing in 1984 that even radical republicans for the most part endorsed conservative corporatist models for understanding women's social roles, an insight that helps to explain why French women gained the vote only in 1945.[26] Other historians have identified the importance of gender-role definitions to legitimizing the republic as a regime obligated to protect and promote the well-being of all its citizenry. Recent studies have demonstrated, for example, that gender politics shaped early welfare policies like family allowances and stood at the center of the pronatalist discourse that underlay much of the republican program.[27] Concern for increasing the nation's birthrate, which had been declining for most of the century, produced a discourse stressing women's primary role as mothers and deploring the effects of female wage work on women's and children's bodies, as well as on men's psyches.

But this emphasis on women's maternal role often clashed directly with the regime's political commitment to establish a secular republican state dedicated to promoting the health and well-being of the population. In France, as in many other European countries, female religious congregations in the nineteenth century provided a vast array of social services; they were teachers, nurses, hospital administrators, apothecaries, welfare administrators, and poor-relief workers. Anticlerical republicans found themselves in a dilemma: if the state was to be responsible for the strength (both collective and individual) of its citizenry, then the provision or at least the regulation of vital social services must lie at the heart of the regime's program. Yet if those services were to be secularized, the state would be forced either to call for the training and employment—at considerable expense—of large numbers of lay women (all potential or actual mothers), or to somehow effect the recoding of social service positions as gender-neutral or even masculine.

In the case of nursing, neither of these solutions sat easily with the republican regime. The first was problematic not only for financial and logistical reasons, but because pronatalist imperatives disinclined republican officials to support the large-scale employment of marriageable women, especially in an unhealthful environment like the hospital. The second ran directly counter to beliefs in women's natural capacity to nurture and to trends within the rapidly organizing medical profession that linked doctors ever more closely with science, which itself was defined as an inherently masculine discipline. Moreover, by the 1880s reformers of all kinds had deemed feminization to be the sine qua non of the modern nursing profession. As the rhetorical link between nursing and religious vocation grew weaker in the heated anticlerical political climate of the period, the association between nursing and essential femininity grew stronger. Even the staunchest advocates of nursing as a skilled medical profession grounded their definitions of the modern nurse in contemporary notions of women's nature.

The continued presence of female congregations in the hospitals allowed the republican administration to avoid facing this insoluble problem. Because the religious sisters existed by definition outside of—even in opposition to—the republican social order, they were to a degree exempt from the regime's gender prescriptions. While for many anticlerical republicans the religious congregations' vow of celibacy was the strongest proof of their members' "unnaturalness," for others the sisterhoods offered a useful way out of a difficult dilemma. By condemning clericalism and the public power of the Church on the one hand, while tolerating active female congregations on the other, republicans could reconcile the secular and gender imperatives of the new political and social order. Even where, as in Lyons, the preservation of bona fide religious congregations proved for various reasons to be impossible, many republicans nonetheless supported a religious model of public hospital nursing.

While contradictions within republican gender imperatives often favored maintaining the status quo regarding hospital nurses, the transformation of the social and medical roles of the hospitals suggested the need for reform.[28] Hospitals in the closing decades of the nineteenth century still served primarily the poor, the old, the abandoned, and the permanently disabled—the outcasts of society. Living conditions in the institutions were barely tolerable. Bed linens were changed infrequently and wards were notoriously filthy. Lying in long rows of metal beds in enormous wards sometimes filled 50 percent above capacity, patients received only marginally edible food (a continual source of dissatisfaction) and were visited irregularly by physicians.[29] In the older institutions (many French hospitals dated back several centuries), temperatures often dipped into the forties during the winter and soared in the summer. Heavy draperies and thick carpets collected dust and germs that were easily transmitted in the crowded wards that grouped together victims of different communicable diseases.[30] Jules Clarétie described Paris's enormous Salpêtrière Hospice for insane women in 1882 as a "sewer where human pain comes to an end . . . It is one of the most somber pages of Parisian life."[31] In the words of one recent historian, the hospitals of the nineteenth century figured "alongside morgues, crime scenes, cemeteries, and the Place de Grève, as one of the primary sites of horror, misery, and suffering."[32] If the schools were the cradle of the republic, the hospitals were still, in the minds of many, its graveyard, reminders of the durability of misery and poverty even in the face of political transformation.

By the close of the century, however, dramatic developments in medical science slowly began to change the abysmal reputation of the hospital. The explosion of experimental research, spurred in large part by the gradual acceptance of the germ theory of disease and the work of Pasteur and Lister, brought international acclaim to the French scientific and medical communities. Although the vast majority of the middle and upper classes continued to receive medical treatment in their homes, a growing percentage of the working class entered the hospital as paying patients. The numbers of non-indigent patients increased rapidly with the passage of the 1898 law on work-related accidents that required employers to pay the medical and pharmaceutical costs for injuries incurred on the job.

By the late 1880s, the government was expending considerable energy promoting the image of public hospitals—at least those that were affiliated with prestigious medical schools and their illustrious faculties—as symbols of the state's concern for the health and not merely the policing of its citizens. In the aftermath of defeat in the Franco-Prussian War of 1870, public officials and social critics of various political stripes sounded the alarm that the French population had lost its vigor and had entered a period of potentially disastrous decline. As a number of historians have shown, this crisis had a strong medical dimension, with contemporary experts pointing to low birth rates and high incidences of infant mortality, tuberculosis, and alcoholism, especially among the poor.[33] Spearheaded by the extraordinary number of physicians who entered the government during this period, medical care became an issue of national political importance. Accordingly, the government established the Conseil Supérieur de l'Assistance Publique in 1888 to organize and oversee the country's various regional programs for free medical care and to advise the Ministry of the Interior on matters pertaining to the nation's health institutions and personnel.[34] The national law on free medical assistance, passed in 1893, stipulated that indigent French citizens (and foreigners with whose government France had a reciprocal agreement) were entitled to medical care at home or in the hospital.[35]

It was within the context of these developments that the reform of hospital nursing emerged for the first time as an issue of national concern in France. Elected officials, physicians, hospital administrators, public health authorities, Church spokespersons, and nurses themselves offered analyses of the strengths and weaknesses of the existing nursing corps in newspapers, journals, speeches, and legislative proposals. In general, the Catholic sisterhoods won accolades from all but the most fanatical anticlerical observers for their selfless dedication to the sick and poor. The nursing sisters, assisted by a growing corps of untrained male and female lay workers, provided all hospital services aside from actual medical care and financial administration. In many large municipal hospitals, the sisters organized and supervised patient care in the wards and oversaw general services such as laundry and food preparation, while the lay employees performed most of the manual labor, including much of the direct patient care. In other institutions, especially smaller ones, nursing sisters provided all secondary hospital services. The nursing sisterhoods enjoyed tremendous popularity in the nineteenth century, especially in rural, undermedicalized areas, where they often supplied the only available health care and social services.

Despite the continuing popularity of the sisters, however, government and health officials grew convinced that the country's existing nursing corps needed considerable reform. Beginning in the 1880s, increasing numbers of observers concerned with the provision of health care asserted that although the ascribed feminine virtues of gentleness, sympathy, tenderness, neatness, docility, devotion, and obedience still constituted the essence of nursing, those attributes no longer sufficed for nurses in a modern hospital. In 1889, the national government issued its first statement of concern that France's hospital nurses had become an anachronism in the era of modern medicine. "Their knowledge is usually purely empirical [meaning 'of empirics, or quacks']," wrote Henri Monod, the national director of Public Assistance, "the most elementary science has no part in it. Too often they lack even the simplest notions of hygiene . . . This defective aspect of hospital organization is becoming increasingly obvious with the progress of medicine and surgery."[36] In 1899 and 1902 the Conseil Supérieur de l'Assistance Publique of the Ministry of the Interior[37] drafted two circulars on the need to reform hospital nursing care, both stressing the need for "true school[s] open to all students wanting to take up a nursing career."[38] Significantly, neither edict mentioned the religious or lay character of any future nursing corps. Indeed, the sole piece of prewar national legislation mandating the establishment of training schools expressly for lay nurses was introduced in the Chamber of Deputies in 1912 and never made it out of committee. Unlike education policy, which centered on guaranteeing the secular character of public schooling, national policy on nursing reform studiously avoided the acrimonious issue altogether. No doubt aware that the merest hint of tendentiousness would elicit cries of treachery from the offended parties (whether clerical or anticlerical), the government chose instead to cast the issue in neutral terms of scientific progress.

The solution to the problem of a deficient nursing corps, the director of the Assistance Publique believed, lay with the government. The state had both the obligation (in accordance with the law of July 15, 1893, guaranteeing medical care to the indigent) and the right (by virtue of its growing financial contribution to medical services) to establish educational standards for the country's nursing personnel.[39] Even supporters of religious nurses, like Lyons hospital administrator Hermann Sabran, admitted that the *congréganistes* were not always "equal to their mission" of providing skilled, hygienic, scientific care in the modern medical age. Sabran blamed an "insufficient professional instruction" for the nurses' increasingly obvious "inferiority."[40]

As for the lay men and women who assisted the *religieuses*, they were almost universally anathematized as ignorant, undisciplined, untrained, unclean, drunken, lazy, and dishonest. Maxime Du Camp, a perennial defender of the nursing sisterhoods, commented that "the [lay] nurses all have the faces of monsters and have remained there [in the hospital] as nurses only because they understand that they could never find a job elsewhere."[41] Recent dramatic scientific advances had further cast existing nursing practices in France in a negative light. While the medical and surgical professions strode boldly into the future, the Conseil Supérieur maintained, nursing remained mired in a premodern era when the public hospital served largely as a haven for the hopeless and helpless—the poor, the elderly, the disabled, and the mentally and mortally ill.[42]

Although doctors were some of the strongest advocates of improved nursing care, their support for full-fledged nursing schools and their graduates was often mitigated by their own professional goals. Spurred by the growing prestige of medical science, doctors initiated an energetic campaign to redefine professional boundaries and solidify authority within the hospitals. Nurses and nursing reformers, struggling to find a place for themselves in the changing hospital environment, frequently found that doctors, their designated collaborators, could also be their fiercest opponents.

A powerful and overwhelmingly left-republican political constituency, physicians were, on the whole, profoundly uncomfortable with the notion of trained female experts on the wards. Doctors' fears that nurses might encroach on their professional terrain arose most directly from their ongoing struggle to defend their field from irregular or illegal practitioners.[43] Until late in the nineteenth century, especially in the countryside, licensed doctors took their place among *officiers de santé* (or second-tier doctors), pharmacists, midwives, local religious orders, and various "empirics" as only one group of experts among many. Although the passage of the 1892 law on medical practice, which (among other things) eliminated the secondary rank of *officiers de santé*, greatly strengthened the doctors' control over the practice of medicine, professional boundaries remained vulnerable. As long as nursing was clearly understood to be a custodial, maternal, or charitable occupation, and as long as the nurses were regarded as the social, economic, and educational peers of the patients, rather than the doctors, there would be no ambiguity about who held medical authority within the hospital.[44] But a more educated and well-trained nurse from a middle-class background could destabilize hierarchies that were just beginning to solidify. Her improved training constituted a potential threat to the doctors' monopoly on medical expertise, and her social status threatened competition over authority in the wards.

It was not for lack of interest or effort that reformers failed to create a corps of trained, secular nurses in France. Far from indifferent, municipal councilmen, hospital administrators, medical practitioners, and nurses' union members in several major cities engaged in heated, at times even vicious, debates over what constituted a proper nurse in the new republic. The multiple images of the public hospital nurse that emerged during this period combined elements of the religious sister with aspects of the domestic worker and of the trained professional, revealing an ongoing conflict over competing and often contradictory definitions of women's roles in the republic.

The history of nursing recounted in this book is, therefore, not in any sense an account of the "rise of the profession," a phrase implying a steady upward climb from obscurity to both popular and official recognition, from subordination to authority, and from formlessness to order. Instead, this work examines the various, often contradictory attempts by government officials of all political stripes, doctors, public health authorities, hospital administrators, and nurses themselves to shape a viable prototype for what I have come to call the "republican nurse." What they ended up with were many different models, which perhaps says as much about the gendered character of the period's social politics and the multiple meanings of female citizenship as it does about the history of nursing itself.

1

Hospital Nursing in Paris

On January 15, 1908, several thousand Parisians, including doctors, municipal councilmen, and national deputies, gathered outside the ancient Hôtel-Dieu Hospital to bid farewell to the Augustine Sisters, the Catholic nursing congregation that had served Paris for nearly a century. The fifty religious women departed in four coaches; the efforts of "a large squadron of police" were required to clear a path for them through the crowd. In a photograph that subsequently appeared in *L'Illustration,* the berobed sisters are barely discernible in the sea of dark overcoats, top hats, and waving white handkerchiefs that overwhelm the waiting carriages.[1] In the context of the controversy that had surrounded the expulsion of the city's religious nurses over the previous thirty years, it is impossible to determine which of these cheering men regretted the sisters' dismissal and which bade them good riddance. What is clear, however, is that the departure of the Augustine Sisters constituted a major event for the city's political and medical elites, an event whose symbolic importance overshadowed concerns about the professional qualifications of the city's nurses. The abrogation of the contract between the city government and the sisters marked the end of three decades of debate that had resulted in the gradual laicization of Paris's public hospital nursing staff. Between 1880 and 1908, proponents of lay nursing engaged in what became at times a fierce struggle with defenders of the religious nursing sisters over both the desired qualities of the hospital nurse and who was best suited to fill that role.

This chapter explores the development of lay hospital nursing in Paris and the social and political forces that informed the various models of "republican nurses" that emerged in the capital city during the three and a half decades before the First World War. As we will see, deeply held beliefs

20

about women's appropriate and natural role in society complicated the otherwise predictable alignment of conservative Catholics behind the sisterhoods and republicans behind lay nursing. It is, in the end, at the intersection of the politics of anticlericalism and the politics of gender that we find the public identity of the municipal hospital nurse in Paris taking shape.

The history of nursing in Paris, as it evolved in the closing decades of the nineteenth century, was inextricably linked to the politics of anticlericalism. Désiré Bourneville's passion for improving the material conditions of the hospital employees' lives and his unflagging promotion of formal training for new and veteran staff alike were deeply rooted in his conviction that all public institutions must be wrested from the influence of the Church. "It is the strict duty of every republican to remove from the priests and the nuns every means of action accorded them in civil society, of which they are the implacable adversaries," Bourneville insisted in 1884. Five years later, frustrated at the pace of laicization, he warned that too many republicans currently in power had forgotten that hospitals and welfare offices *(bureaux de bienfaisance)* were "the homes of fanaticism and counter-revolution."[2]

Bourneville's conceptualization of a society threatened at its very core by its reliance on the services of religious functionaries was hardly remarkable in the 1880s, the heyday of republican anticlerical fervor. Under the leadership of such men as Léon Gambetta and Jules Ferry, the newly secure republican government quickly passed a series of laws aimed at reducing and later eliminating Church influence in public education.[3] Bourneville, who served on the Paris Municipal Council from 1876 to 1883 and in the Chamber of Deputies from 1883 to 1890, maintained that Church control in the wards of the city's hospitals presented no less of a threat to the future of the republic than did the presence of nuns and Jesuits in the primary schools.[4]

Unlike in the schools, however, the danger in the hospitals arose less from the direct influence of the Catholic sisters over vulnerable members of the population than from the potent and subversive presence in public institutions of a personnel that recognized an authority outside the control of the state. The very existence of an autonomous community of women called into question the hierarchy of power within municipal institutions. Because these women looked to the Church for direction, their presence constituted a concrete political threat to secular authority. "The character of the congregational personnel does not allow for direct communication with the administrative authority," observed Charles Quentin, the director of the Assistance Publique, "because the observations that the sisters gather are first transmitted, not to the directors, but to the superiors of the orders . . . With the congregational element the administration is not the sole mistress in its own home."[5] The religious congregations were, as one historian has remarked, a "state within a state" and thus a threat to legitimate national authority.[6]

Notably absent from much of the political discourse on the laicization of the Parisian hospitals were accusations of intolerance on the part of the sisters, one of the most common criticisms of the country's active religious orders.[7] Proponents of laicization occasionally complained about proselytizing, unequal treatment of patients, and neglect of duty resulting from religious obligations, but the charges were usually invoked only to counter claims of lay nurses' incompetence. The relative lack of interest in the sisters' behavior stemmed, in large part, from the minimal amount of direct contact between the religious nurses and the patients. Employed exclusively as *surveillantes,* or head nurses, the sisters served in a supervisory capacity, maintaining discipline, organizing the distribution of food, and overseeing the changing of dressings and the administration of various treatments. The bulk of the actual patient care was performed by lay *infirmières* and *infirmiers,* or even by *filles de service,* a point that the supporters of laicization did not hesitate to use against the sisters. "It must be said once and for all that the sisters have never cared for patients in either the medical or the surgical wards," insisted one anticlerical member of the municipal council. The lay *infirmières* and *infirmiers,* not the sisters, prepared and administered dressings and poultices.[8] If the sisters did not actually provide care for the patients, he asked, then on what basis, short of the overtly political, could anyone argue for retaining the nuns in the wards? The qualities of sympathy and self-abnegation, touted as the special strength of the sisters, were hardly required of supervisory nurses.

By 1880, the first round of hospital laicization in Paris had been completed and, according to the proponents of secular nursing, had proved to be successful. Yet the terms by which administrators evaluated that success were revealing. Charles Quentin observed that in all four institutions, Laennec, Lenoir-Trousseau, La Pitié, and Les Tournelles, the smooth functioning of services "left nothing to be desired." He noted, in particular, that the secular authorities in the hospitals now exercised full control over the new nurses. A medical inspector at the Laennec Hospital similarly reported that the new lay personnel had the great advantage of being "infinitely more subordinate than the religious nurses and more scrupulous in the strict execution of the doctors' orders."[9] The director of the hospice Les Tournelles agreed that the lay personnel there was, above all, more compliant with the authority of both the medical staff and the hospital administration. The *surveillantes,* he observed, "submit much more easily . . . to the pressure of the medical corps . . . From an administrative and disciplinary point of view . . . their obedience to the administration to which they report is assured." The chain of command had crystallized: directors of the hospitals had established clear control over the new supervisory staff, and the lay *surveillantes* and *surveillants* had themselves managed to assert their authority over the subordinate staff.[10]

The laicizations of 1878–1880 aroused little substantial popular or political opposition, primarily because the replacement of the religious sisters coincided with other changes that made the abrogation of the contracts with the congregations appear less overtly political. The Laennec Hospital, for example, had served as a temporary facility for years. The laicization of its supervisory nursing staff became part of the institution's general transformation into a permanent hospital. Sweeping personnel changes accompanied the reorganization of services and attracted little public attention. In the case of La Pitié, the superior of the Sisters of Sainte-Marthe had herself, in July 1880, requested the termination of the congregation's contract with the city of Paris, citing the difficulty of maintaining recruitment levels. Désiré Bourneville praised the Sisters of Sainte-Marthe as "the most devoted and most tolerant of the nursing orders," and stressed that it was the Jesuits' condemnation of the order as too "independent" that led to its downfall. The municipal council could thus cast the laicization of La Pitié as the product of intolerance within the Church.[11]

The rash of anticlerical laws passed in the early 1880s enabled the council to claim further that the laicization of Paris hospital staffs was part of a broad national program to regulate religious orders and limit their presence in public institutions. In March 1880 the national government had issued a decree requiring all non-authorized religious orders to apply for official recognition within three months, and in June the Jesuits were expelled from the country. In early 1881, the Conseil de Surveillance, which oversaw the administration of all institutions of the Assistance Publique, voted unanimously (with one abstention) for the laicization of all hospices, hospitals, and *maisons de secours* (private hospitals) in the Department of the Seine. By the spring of that year, four more institutions had been laicized, and one more in the spring of 1882.[12] Yet by the middle of the decade, when Bourneville left his seat on the Paris Municipal Council to serve in the Chamber of Deputies, the pace slowed dramatically. Nearly half the hospitals, hospices, and foundations administered by the Assistance Publique (thirteen out of twenty-seven) still employed religious *surveillantes* by the summer of 1884.[13]

In contrast to the hospital laicizations of 1878–1880, the aggressive campaign of 1881–1884 to secularize nursing in all Parisian public hospitals aroused vocal opposition almost from the outset. Clerical and politically conservative journals like *La Nouvelliste*, *La Croix*, and *Le Journal des débats* printed predictable, almost formulaic articles praising the virtue and devotion of the religious sisters and condemning the venality and ineptitude of their lay replacements. To the anticlerical members of the municipal council and the Assistance Publique administration, articles such as these could only have strengthened their claim that continued support for the nursing orders was primarily politically motivated.

Far more problematic than the unsurprising conservative defense of the sisters were the strong objections to laicization leveled by a heavily republican, often left-leaning constituency in the hospitals—the doctors. In March 1881 five doctors and a surgeon from the as yet unlaicized Tenon Hospital protested to the director general of the Assistance Publique against the administration's recent resolution supporting the complete laicization of all AP institutions. The physicians' complaints were twofold: first, they claimed that they had not been consulted in the decision to replace the sisters. Second, and more important, they found no reason to replace competent and devoted nurses: "The sisters have proved themselves; we have witnessed their devotion to the patients, the order that they maintain in the wards. We do not know who will replace them. The eviction of the sisters would thus be an act of imprudence and ingratitude."[14]

The Tenon letter was widely dismissed by proponents of laicization on the grounds that its authors had no experience working with lay *surveillantes*. But the same could not be said of the missive that arrived at the director general's office two days later. Sixty doctors and surgeons from every nonlaicized institution and several laicized ones signed a brief letter attesting to the competence and character of the religious sisters. "Considering the question from the sole point of view of the benefit to the service and the interests of the patients," the document stated simply, "we are convinced that the system currently in practice is preferable to that which would replace it." The signatories, who grew in number to eighty-four within a few days, objected to what they perceived to be a misguided politicization of the administrative function of the Assistance Publique and a blatant lack of consideration for the best interests of the doctors and their patients.[15] The religious orders' emphasis on obedience, discipline, and self-abnegating devotion undoubtedly appealed greatly to physicians still uncertain of their authority within the hospitals. Dr. Anger, a surgeon at Beaujon, noted that "women who have been regimented and disciplined as were the nuns would be easier to handle for the management."[16] More-over, the sisters, though many came from lower-class backgrounds, stood apart from the patients and the lower-level personnel by their dress, their daily prayer schedule, and their existence as an autonomous organization under contract—but not subordinate—to the Assistance Publique admin-istration. The religious *surveillantes* thus maintained a natural authority over their patients without presenting a threat to the doctors' control in the medical sphere.

It is also not improbable that some physicians found the sisters' presence in the wards to be useful in persuading patients of the efficacy of medical therapies. Even in the late nineteenth century, much of the public re-mained unconvinced of the healing capacity of formally trained doctors, and many still put their faith in unlicensed practitioners. In rural areas in particular, religious congregations often served as the chief—and in some cases the only—source of medical services and pharmaceutical supplies. As Ralph Gibson has recently observed, the congregations "were operating in a society where biological suffering and the Catholic faith were still seen as intimately related . . . They were prepared to take on the repulsive, the in-curable, and the financially unrewarding in a way that doctors were often not."[17] However pragmatic or even self-serving the physicians' motives were, it is clear that many of them saw no contradiction between the prin-ciple of scientific medical progress and the persistence of religious nursing care. When, for example, the Pasteur Institute director Dr. Emile Roux and his colleague Dr. Louis Martin established the Pasteur Hospital in 1900, they turned to the Sisters of Saint-Joseph-de-Cluny to staff their wards precisely because, according to one recruit, the doctors felt it would be easy "to train them in the new Pasteurian methods."[18]

Doctors' opposition to secularization peaked in the 1880s and 1890s with the remarkable efforts of the surgeon Armand Desprès, who, for a decade and a half, ran a tireless propaganda campaign on behalf of the Catholic nursing orders. Immediately in the wake of the Conseil de Surveillance's February 1881 vote to laicize all AP institutions, Desprès began what would become a decade-long struggle against the majority opinion in the municipal council on which he served from 1884 to 1889. In numerous letters to newspapers and journals (most notably the *Gazette des hôpitaux*), as well as in impassioned speeches in the municipal council and Chamber of Deputies (to which he was elected in 1889), Desprès argued that nursing was "the natural occupation of the nun," and that lay women were incapable of the sort of selfless devotion to the helpless that the position required. Desprès's ongoing debate with his fellow doctor-politician Bourneville over the merits and deficiencies of religious and lay nurses grew so hostile that at one point it allegedly almost led to a duel.[19]

Over the course of the 1880s and early 1890s, Desprès's name became virtually synonymous with the effort to return the nuns to the hospitals (in common parlance, the *reintégration*). But the majority within the municipal council remained unconvinced and grew increasingly impatient with the eccentric surgeon. By the time he was elected to the Chamber of Deputies in 1889, his longwinded and predictable speeches elicited mostly dismissive responses.[20] Desprès died in 1896, having witnessed the laicization of all but two Parisian hospitals and five private foundations.

The ultimate failure of his campaign notwithstanding, what distinguishes Desprès's defense of the sisters from the numerous other pleas on behalf of religious nursing is that he predicated his position on his identity as a staunch, anticlerical republican. Desprès, who like Bourneville called himself a Freethinker, arrived on the political scene in 1876 when he led the opposition to a new administrative measure that would require every hospital patient's bed to display a card noting the occupant's religious affiliation. Throughout his career, Desprès never ceased to deplore religious proselytizing nor hesitated to label Catholicism an "oppressive religion."[21] Despite his consistent hostility to the Church, Desprès insisted that "if it were not for the need to guard against proselytism at the patient's bedside, the religious nursing sister would be . . . the ideal of perfection." He reasoned that since it was the clergy that forced the nursing sisters to proselytize among the patients, there was no reason to dismiss the religious nurses.[22] The political goal of republican anticlericalism must remain limited to the destruction of the clergy as a political force. Moreover, the surgeon warned, the campaign to remove the religious sisters from the hospitals could well backfire for republicans, for if the lay nurses proved to be incompetent, the entire anticlerical project might founder. Not only did the French countryside remain deeply religious, Desprès maintained, but tens of thousands of republicans in Paris alone had voted for reactionary candidates in protest against the republican politicians' attacks on the sisters. The key to winning their votes lay in preserving the nursing sisterhoods.[23]

Political pragmatism aside, what Desprès's diatribes expressed (albeit at times in extreme form) was the widespread republican ambivalence about lay women's role in public hospitals. Desprès's case for maintaining the Catholic sisters rested not on any great love for the nuns—Desprès himself came from a Protestant family—but on his conviction that nursing was fundamentally incompatible with the lives of lay women. The first obligation of every woman not affiliated with a religious order, he argued, was to her private family and household. If her husband or child fell ill, she would, as a good wife and mother, abandon her patients, and might even be tempted to steal food from the hospital to feed her family. The lay nurse also risked infecting her family with diseases contracted in the wards.[24] The sisters made ideal nurses precisely because they were women by nature, but without the attributes of womanhood that society conferred. "A woman is either a bad mother or a bad nurse," Desprès wrote in 1886. "Under [the nun's] headdress is a woman, a woman who sacrifices everything that gives joy to other women and devotes herself to the repugnant task of being continuously with the sick."[25] Because the nuns had no families of their own, they alone could serve as surrogate mothers to the ill and impoverished patients who populated turn-of-the-century hospital wards.

In contrast to the lay nurse, the nursing sister had no children but her patients, no home but the hospital. The religious nurse, according to Desprès, was "a woman who has neither family nor pecuniary interests, who no longer even has a name and who calls herself 'sister,' who lives the life of a prisoner, who sleeps in a dormitory, eats the same food as the patients in a refectory, and who, 365 days a year, from four in the morning until ten at night . . . can give her time to the patients with clockwork regularity."[26] Desprès's colleague Dr. Potain concurred, noting that "for the nursing sister, her life interest is completely contained in the ward for which she is responsible. That is her home." The nursing sister sacrificed her family, her comfort, even her own name, for the benefit of anonymous others. Nursing was not a displacement or transference of women's maternal instinct, but a duty so onerous and so noxious that only "an impersonal being" could perform it properly.[27]

Després's line of argument, though largely polemical in intent, was part of a broader debate about the relationship of nursing to women's role in society. The identification of hospital nursing as an essentially feminine occupation predated by centuries the foundation of the numerous female nursing orders in the seventeenth century. But the belief that women *alone* were capable of tending the sick in the wards was of much more recent vintage. Even in 1900, more than a quarter of the upper-level nursing positions and more than half of the lower-level jobs in the municipal hospitals of Paris were held by men.[28] Bourneville claimed that he first became convinced of the principle of feminization in 1877, and it was only two years later that he successfully argued in favor of a resolution in the municipal council urging the Assistance Publique administration to replace men with women wherever possible.[29] Five years later Bourneville announced his intention to feminize all nursing positions in Paris hospitals that involved patient care on the wards.[30]

By the mid-1890s government authorities had accepted the feminization of hospital nursing, at least in principle. An inspector for the Assistance Publique noted that the move toward feminization was a "natural trend," given women's "delicate hand," "tender sympathy," and talent for finding words of consolation. Henri Napias, hospital inspector for the Ministry of the Interior (and later director of the AP administration), pointed to the success of the English model as proof of women's innate capacity for superior nursing. "The English have understood that caring for the sick belongs especially to women; they alone have the qualities of gentleness . . . grace and charm that are indispensable to the task . . . The hospital is a big house of which they are the informed housewives and managers."[31] A year later, the Conseil Supérieur de l'Assistance Publique began devising a blueprint for nursing schools throughout the country grounded on the principle that "from the point of view of patient care as well as economy and orderliness, the presence of women should be preferred."[32] The Ministry of the Interior's 1899 circular on the recruitment and training of nurses based on that blueprint insisted that women made superior nurses and were to be favored over men for most positions involving patient care.

In contrast to Després, who believed that maternity disqualified lay women from nursing, many proponents of laicization argued that it was precisely the experience of motherhood and domesticity and the character traits that those roles drew upon that suited women to nursing. Women's monopoly over the capacity to provide sympathetic and effective care resonated deeply in a society increasingly alarmed by the nation's low birth rate and obsessed with the connection between maternal behavior and infant mortality rates. The rhetoric of the maternal and domestic roots of nursing thus effectively harnessed the broad political consensus around pronatalism to the laicization process. Dr. Julien Noir, a frequent contributor to *Le Progrès médical*, went so far as to consider all women who chose celibacy to be the moral and political equivalent of members of a religious order. Denouncing the English model of accepting only single, educated, young women as nurses, Noir stated in 1905 that "we want them to be married, even mothers because some of the tenderness of feeling for the weak and for the children only flower fully in the heart of a mother."[33] Noir believed that the hospital was, in essence, a household that required a woman's presence to insure both its benevolent character and efficient functioning. Hence only married women could be entrusted with the responsibility of running the hospital wards, because they alone were fully women. Whereas to Desprès nursing and domestic womanhood were incompatible because each constituted a complete identity that brooked no competition, to Noir, Bourneville, and the vast majority of the supporters of laicization, nursing and domesticity were simply different aspects of an essential, female identity. Ironically, Desprès's line of reasoning would find its clearest echo in the reform efforts of Anna Hamilton, who stressed celibacy as a prerequisite for a full-fledged nursing career.

In the end, Desprès's vision of the nurse who, in the name of service, sacrificed "everything that gives joy to other women," along with a salary and an independent life, failed to gain ascendance in Paris. When he died in 1896, only one nursing order remained in service in the municipal hospitals: the Augustine Sisters of the Hôtel-Dieu and the Hôpital Saint-Louis, who would remain for another decade. Finally, in 1906, the government issued the required decree abrogating the city's contract with its last surviving nursing congregation. On January 15, 1908, the Augustine Sisters withdrew to the private Hôpital Notre-Dame de Bon-Secours, which from then on would serve as the Maison-Mère of the order. Just over a year later, in May 1909, Désiré Bourneville died. An era had drawn to a close.[34] The Parisian laicization project weathered one final challenge in 1913, when a more conservative municipal council began to push for *reintégration.* The onset of war eight months later, however, brought all plans for further hospital reform to a halt.[35]

From the beginning of the municipal council's laicization campaign in the late 1870s, advocates recognized that the project's success depended on demonstrating that laywomen and men (and later laywomen alone) were more competent and more knowledgeable than the religious sisters. Opponents of the nursing congregations never tired of describing the sisters' limitations: as members of a religious order, their primary concern was for the spiritual rather than physical health of the patient; their revulsion against all matters of the flesh made them resistant to modern hygiene measures and new antiseptic techniques. Most orders prohibited their members from viewing naked men, or, in the case of the Daughters of Charity of Saint-Vincent de Paul, from diapering male infants. All were forbidden to care for women in childbirth, and some could not treat single mothers. Finally, the proponents of laicization argued that all claims that the *religieuses* were the cheapest form of hospital labor were misleading, because their limitations forced the institutions to hire extra personnel to perform duties that the sisters abjured. The religious nurses were categorically incapable of becoming the enlightened doctors' assistants that modern medical science required and that so many other countries already had.[36]

But who would replace the sisters? Removing the *religieuses* was a purely political challenge, but finding competent replacements for them was a much more complicated problem. Even the most enthusiastic advocates of laicization acknowledged that the existing lay staff, including those who served in the wards, was woefully deficient. "The lay secondary personnel of the hospitals and hospices is almost always recruited from among the illiterate class," noted Assistance Publique Director Charles Quentin in 1880, and was "a stranger to the most elementary ideas and to professional knowledge of hospital service."[37]

Even Bourneville admitted that the existing lay personnel was drastically undereducated and undertrained. He once described the Salpêtrière Hospice, which had always had a lay staff, as a refuge for young girls from notoriously school-deficient Brittany and Savoie who "come to Paris seeking a better life."[38] In 1878 Bourneville warned that laicization would fail unless the city government set up professional training classes for the secular staff. Already the Conseil de Surveillance had rejected a proposal to laicize one hospital on the grounds that absent a nursing school, "no other institution (except the religious orders) could furnish a personnel with the same guarantees of aptitude and devotion."[39] Without a training school for lay nurses, Bourneville and his colleagues could not defend their project; without a school, there would be no personnel capable of filling the vacant positions.

The nursing schools that opened in two Parisian hospitals in the spring of 1878—one for women (*infirmières*) at the Salpêtrière and one for men (*infirmiers*) at Bicêtre[40]—were hardly the professional training programs that Bourneville and Quentin had hoped for. Instead, both institutions initially offered only hour-long classes, three times a week, in basic reading, writing, and arithmetic. The introduction of primary schooling into the hospitals filled an urgent need to provide a basic education to the large number of staff members who entered service with essentially no schooling. All forty-five of the women who showed up for the first primary school class at the Salpêtrière were illiterate.[41] A decade later, Bourneville noted that of the 843 women who had attended the Salpêtrière primary school since its opening, 343 (over 40%) had been illiterate or nearly illiterate. Even in 1889, a full quarter of the 280 who took primary school classes at the Salpêtrière could neither read nor write. Not before the 1905–06 academic year could the school claim an entering class without a single illiterate student.[42]

The full proposal for France's first public professional training program for nurses, issued by the Assistance Publique administration in November 1880, called for the creation of primary schools for employees in each of the city's thirteen major institutions. Instruction would consist of five- or six-week long courses in elementary reading, writing, arithmetic, and geography, as well as "basic professional" skills. The latter would include lessons on the organization and administration of the hospitals, basic anatomy and physiology, and fundamental techniques of minor surgery, dressings, bandages, baths, and other treatments.[43]

The centerpiece of the professional training program was the advanced courses that were to be set up in the Salpêtrière and Bicêtre Hospices for the most promising candidates. Based explicitly on the model provided by the English nursing schools, the Paris program combined classroom lectures by medical personnel with practical exercises led by some of the more experienced *surveillantes*.[44] Like their counterparts in England, students were to be assigned a special dormitory with its own dining facility, and a "study room, classroom, and common room" apart from the rest of the institution. Unlike in England, however, students in Paris would play no direct role in the daily functioning of the hospitals. Their experience on the wards was to be limited to observing the doctors' and interns' rounds and to substituting in the various services during the vacation period. At the end of a year, students who passed a juried exam would enter the hospital staff at the level of second-class *infirmière* or *infirmier*, or first class *fille* or *garçon de service*.[45]

The program that the Assistance Publique administration actually established in the two hospitals fell far short of the original plan. While the primary school sessions were lengthened to two hours, the professional courses met only once a week for one hour. Practical training remained limited to brief rotations in the general infirmary, where groups of ten students at a time would "assist in dressing blisters, bedsores, ulcers, in applying cupping-glasses, leeches, etc." Those in the most advanced courses spent a maximum of fifteen days in the general services assisting, for example, in the kitchen or the laundry.[46]

In 1880, on Bourneville's suggestion, the Assistance Publique opened a third professional school at La Pitié Hospital as an *école de perfectionnement* for exceptionally capable students seeking more advanced and specialized training. Unlike Salpêtrière and Bicêtre, which served primarily as hospices for the indigent elderly and mentally ill, La Pitié offered a wide range of medical specialties, including obstetrics, services for the treatment of specific acute illnesses, and a large surgery department. Bourneville and the AP administration quickly recognized, however, that the existing personnel of La Pitié, like their colleagues in Salpêtrière and Bicêtre, lacked even the most basic skills.[47] Forced to adjust the curriculum to focus on reading and arithmetic, Bourneville never succeeded in turning the Pitié school into an *école de perfectionnement,* despite repeated efforts throughout the late 1880s and 1890s.

The first years of the schools' operation were marked by low enrolments and high attrition rates. Perpetually frustrated at the slow pace of laicization, Bourneville was particularly concerned about the failure of the upper-level or *gradé* personnel (*surveillantes, sous-surveillantes,* and *suppléantes*) to attend classes in substantial numbers. After all, the administration relied upon this group to replace the nursing sisters in laicized hospitals. In 1882–83, for example, not a single *sous-surveillante* at the

Salpêtrière participated in the practical exams, and only a few *suppléantes* took the written test at the end of the year. In 1890 only one member of the *personnel gradé* of La Pitié received a diploma.[48]

As the number of laicized institutions multiplied in the mid-1880s, the supply of competent nurses with the experience and skills necessary to serve as *surveillantes* declined steadily. Bourneville recognized that unless the schools actively recruited educated women from outside the existing hospital staffs, the administration would be forced to hire incompetent or untrained nurses. This would have potentially disastrous implications for the laicization project. Hoping to attract unemployed teachers to the hospitals, he made a special appeal to women "who have occupied a more or less high position in the world and have fallen from fortune or comfort into a precarious situation." But the educated women that he sought to attract never materialized. French women, Bourneville lamented in 1896, still had not grasped the importance of nursing training for all women. The country still lagged far behind England where, he maintained, even rich young girls attended classes and served in the hospitals.[49]

The recruitment efforts were not in vain, however, and the attendance problems proved short-lived. By the early 1890s about half the upper-level nursing staff in all Parisian municipal hospitals had received diplomas, and a decade later that figure had risen to two-thirds. By the mid-1890s the pace of laicizations had slowed, and there was no shortage of nursing staff with diplomas.[50] Much to Bourneville's disappointment, however, the growing numbers of nurses with professional degrees did not translate into a better educated staff. Enthusiasm for the diploma, which often led to faster promotions for its recipients, far outstripped the employees' desire for a *certificat d'études* signifying mastery of a basic elementary education. At the turn of the century, two-thirds of the top four ranks of personnel had received diplomas, while at most one quarter had any type of educational degree (from the most basic *certificat d'études élémentaires* on up).[51] Bourneville himself complained that "in Paris the Public Assistance administration is forced to accept women who, far from having an [elementary] certificate, often have a rudimentary primary education." Prospective nurses, Bourneville insisted, should be required to have at least the same amount of education as those who apply for jobs in workshops or businesses.[52]

Bourneville's exhortations notwithstanding, nurses and other hospital employees had little incentive to devote precious hours to primary education. Although nurses with diplomas were occasionally denied promotions on the grounds of inadequate primary education, lower-level workers were far more likely to be passed over if they had no nursing diploma than if they were deficient in reading, writing, or arithmetic.[53] With fourteen- or fifteen-hour work days, few nurses had either the time or the energy to take multiple evening classes. Forced to choose between a primary degree, which in and of itself brought no material benefits, and a professional diploma that might increase their chances for promotion, most opted for the latter.

From the perspective of those who supported the rapid replacement of the religious sisters by lay personnel, the Paris municipal nursing school programs were, on balance, a success. What better way to demonstrate to the skeptical public the competence of the lay nurses than by citing the ever-expanding number of "professionals" among them? For the degree recipients themselves, however, the professional advantages of the diploma were becoming increasingly less apparent. By the 1890s many graduates found that even professional degrees brought them no substantive rewards. Although most, if not all, promotions were granted to nurses with diplomas, there simply were not enough promotions to go around. Bourneville and other doctors who taught in the nursing schools began urging graduates to seek employment outside Paris, in newly laicized hospitals in the provinces or even in private hospitals and homes.[54]

The excessive number of nursing diplomas distributed in Paris elicited criticism from both inside and outside the institutions. One *surveillante* accused the administration of granting diplomas indiscriminately in order to inflate statistics and make the lay nursing staff appear more competent than it actually was. "Linen maids, laundresses, autopsy assistants," none of whom provided patient care, attended the schools. "Everyone is given a diploma," she complained, "even those who receive below average grades from the professor. . . . There are those who work . . . and deserve their diploma. But [the diploma] no longer has any value if everyone gets one."[55] Municipal council member Edmond Lepelletier, noting the "rudimentary" character of the instruction offered in the schools, deemed the yearly increases in the number of diplomas issued "a veritable trompe-l'oeil that serves only to deceive the municipal council and the Paris population."[56] By 1905, with the Paris schools granting over 400 diplomas annually, the Assistance Publique administration instituted more stringent examination standards in an effort to stem the devaluation of the degree. Only those who demonstrated mastery of real knowledge and skills should receive an official diploma.[57] Within two years the number of degrees issued fell to 262, and by 1909 it dropped to 186.

Bourneville's municipal nursing schools came under attack not just for the alleged worthlessness of the training and degrees they provided, but also, ironically, for the excessive scientific content of their theoretical courses. This apparent contradiction betrayed a widespread uncertainty about the role of the modern lay nurse: was she to be a lay replacement for the religious sister, providing care and consolation out of a sense of charity and maternal sympathy? Was she to be a female laborer, from a working-class or peasant background, trained formally and through experience in some basic nursing techniques? Or was she to be a full-fledged professional, schooled in a medical specialty suited to feminine talents? The latter possibility clearly elicited anxiety among the policy-makers of the Conseil Supérieur de l'Assistance Publique, revealing the government's mistrust of nursing as a true profession. In its 1899 national nursing reform program, the CSAP pointedly refused to adopt Bourneville's training programs as a model on the grounds that they were "too theoretical," and that their emphasis on classroom knowledge over practical expertise tempted students "to take initiative that belongs to the doctor alone."[58] The CSAP's plan, which was sent to all the departments in 1902, advocated instead a one-year program that focused almost exclusively on training in the wards and reduced to an absolute minimum the amount of time spent studying such subjects as anatomy and physiology. Nursing, the planners suggested, was essentially a vocation best learned through practice and experience. Any attempts to convert it into a medical profession were dangerously misguided.

Because Bourneville's nursing schools were so explicitly tied to the laicization project, they were also vulnerable to political criticism. Throughout the first two decades of the schools' existence, Bourneville and his supporters (and, at times, the Assistance Publique director) persistently stressed the lay nurses' usefulness in solidifying the Third Republic. By educating and granting degrees to the "valiant daughters of the people," Paris furnished the nation with a veritable female army of soldiers for the nation.[59] But the schools' high political profile could also become a liability when the political climate changed. In 1900, in the midst of the Dreyfus Affair, Parisians elected a majority of nationalists to the municipal council.[60] In the summer following the election, councilman Edmond

Lepelletier, an anticlerical member of the Ligue de la Libre Pensée and a fervent anti-Dreyfusard, launched a broad attack on the schools, citing the incompetence of the instructors and the general inadequacy of the courses. The real target of his criticism, however, was not the substance of the training program but the politicization of the institutions. Lepelletier argued that Bourneville had turned the training facilities into partisan camps, using the annual awards ceremonies as vehicles for disseminating Dreyfusard propaganda. "I do not want Dreyfusism to get publicity in the hospitals," he declared, amid cries of "very good! very good!" from the council. "I am attacking M. Bourneville because he is marching with the enemies of the country and the Republic." In an effort to reduce political tensions, the AP director decided that the ceremonies would henceforth be open only to faculty and students, and that only the hospital director (and thus not Bourneville) would be allowed to deliver a brief speech appropriate to the occasion. [61]

But those restrictions did not satisfy the Paris Municipal Council, determined as it was to wrest control of the schools from Bourneville. In November 1900, the council voted to eliminate the budget for the existing schools and to create, instead, new courses under its own auspices.[62] The resolution did not have the effect intended by Lepelletier and his backers. Within three weeks of its passage, the professors at the schools submitted a letter to the director of Assistance Publique pledging their services without salary. In February of 1901 the Prefect of the Seine declared the Paris Municipal Council's resolution illegal on the grounds that it overstepped the authority of the city government.[63] In the end, Bourneville and the nursing school instructors got more political mileage out of the resolution than did its sponsors. Casting himself as the victim of an authoritarian and censorious political cabal and the faculty as selfless public servants, Bourneville and the schools emerged from the brief crisis with strong political support in the Dreyfusard press and in the national government.

Although the political threat to laicization subsided with the passage of the law on associations in 1901, the need to reform hospital nursing and lift it above the status of domestic work persisted. Already in 1898, inspector Henri Napias had documented in discouraging detail the inferiority of France's nursing corps to that of the United States and several European countries. Napias attributed the disparity to the overall failure of the French hospitals to attract the type of candidate required to transform nursing from a form of domestic service to a bona fide women's profession. Among the most obvious causes were the meager salaries accorded lay hospital nurses in France. The administration "tries above all to spend as little as possible on the personnel," he asserted. "The nurses are given a salary that is almost always, if not always, lower than that of an ordinary domestic servant."[64] The *Revue philanthropique,* mouthpiece of the Assistance Publique administration, likewise compared the nurse's wages to those of a "general servant." Low pay, combined with the requirement that the nurses sleep in dormitories, "deters from the hospitals those who would most enhance the reputation of the nursing profession."[65] The AP director observed that even the best nurses "were disgusted by an occupation whose onerous and repugnant character is not compensated by any benefits."[66] If French hospitals were to meet the challenges presented by the other European countries and by the advances of medical science, administrators and politicians would have to take clear steps toward establishing nursing as, at the very least, a skilled occupation, if not a prestigious career.

Although Napias's report was aimed principally at the need for reform in provincial cities and towns, the Assistance Publique administration and Bourneville himself recognized that in Paris too the existing system had reached the limits of its potential for improvement. Without dramatic changes in training programs and the organization of nursing work, as well as in the material conditions of employment, nursing in Paris would remain essentially a form of domestic service. The key to the reform of nursing, Bourneville now insisted, no longer lay solely in transforming the poor, uneducated, and untrained "daughters of the people" into skilled and efficient "soldiers of the Republic." Returning to the position he had adopted—without success—in the mid-1880s, Bourneville once again argued that the future of the profession depended on attracting educated women who already had a sense of public mission and who found in the hospitals an attractive venue in which to exercise their talents. Bourneville predicted in 1900 that "serious, worthy, educated women will only consent to offer their services to the sick if they are guaranteed a little consideration and suitable, healthful material conditions."[67] Given the proper moral and material assurances, the *Revue philanthropique* concurred, thousands of educated women in Paris would eagerly enter nursing. After all, approximately 9,000 educated young women had recently applied for teaching positions in primary or nursery schools in the Department of the Seine, and fifteen or twenty thousand were seeking employment in banks or department stores.[68] Somehow, the AP administrators had to refashion hospital nursing into a viable career alternative for this select group of women.

The most obvious obstacle to achieving this goal was the appalling conditions in which the nursing staff was forced to work and live. Most nurses slept in crowded, dingy dormitories that were virtual incubators of disease. "The access corridors, the walls, the doors, the windows, are all poorly cleaned, disgusting," Bourneville said of the Lariboisière Hospital in 1896. "One wonders when was the last time there had been a serious cleaning."[69] Assistance Publique Director Charles Mourier noted in 1902 that after a fourteen- or fifteen-hour work day, nurses retired to "dormitories . . . where the beds touch one another, where there is no air, where one freezes in winter and where in summer a terrible heat reigns . . . there are no washstands, no water-closets, and everyone lives in a state of promiscuity in which morals often suffer and where all sense of personal dignity is dulled."[70] If the administration wanted to attract educated young women to the staff, the hospitals had to provide decent living quarters.

The deplorable housing situation only compounded the physical dangers posed by hazardous conditions in the wards themselves. One member of the Conseil de Surveillance described the work places of hospital nurses as "more unhealthful than those in which certain industrial workers labor, places that are fortunately slated for disappearance in the near future." Even a healthy woman who entered hospital service stood a very good chance of contracting a life-threatening illness, either from a patient or from a co-worker. Between May 1895 and May 1896, the support personnel of all Paris hospitals suffered a thirteen-percent mortality rate. Forty percent of those deaths were attributed to tuberculosis.[71] To make matters worse, these figures included only those who died while employed by the hospital and did not take into account the untold numbers that left the institution for health reasons and died at home or elsewhere. The incidence of tuberculosis among the nursing staff was so high that in 1903 the Assistance Publique administration explicitly excluded the disease from the list of illnesses for which employees could receive monetary compensation, on the grounds that it simply could not afford the enormous expense.[72]

Despite compelling evidence pointing to the need for material improvements, the 1903 hospital regulations devised by an AP-appointed committee of health administrators focused almost exclusively on organizational reforms. The director of the Assistance Publique admitted regretfully (and much to the dismay of the increasingly vocal employees' associations) that financial constraints imposed by the Paris Municipal Council made it impossible to institute significant salary increases or large-scale improvements in housing or food quality. Instead, the proposed reforms advanced three fundamental goals which, when attained, would ostensibly transform nursing in Paris into a respectable women's profession with a clear place in the occupational hierarchy of the hospital. First, the regulations redefined nursing as skilled, direct patient care, distinct from work in such general services as the hospital laundry or kitchen. Second, they mandated the feminization of all nursing positions involving direct patient care. In the future, men would be employed as caregiving nurses (*soignants*) only in special wards considered unsuitable for women, namely those that treated men with venereal diseases or urinary tract conditions. Third, the new guidelines stressed the absolute necessity of a rigorous, full-time, two-year nursing school whose graduates would, over time, comprise the entire nursing staff of the Parisian hospitals.

The first of these tenets addressed directly the problem of job definition that had plagued efforts to boost the professional status of hospital work in Paris for over twenty-five years. A woman or man, trained or untrained, could (and often did) serve interchangeably in the sick wards and in general services. This practice had several adverse repercussions. It meant, for example, that a *première infirmière* (the highest rank in the *non-gradé* category of employment) who cared for patients in the sick wards drew the same salary and was accorded the same professional status as a *première infirmière* working in the laundry room. Likewise, the titles *infirmière* and *surveillante*, as well as the intermediary ranks of *suppléante* and *sous-surveillante*, were not attached to a set of skills and responsibilities and thus had no specific professional identities. They were all simply hierarchical ranks within the mass of hospital secondary personnel.

For the individual employee, the lack of professional differentiation between ward nursing and general services had the effect of inhibiting specialization and rendering personal preferences or aptitudes irrelevant. Because salaries in the hospitals were allocated according to rank, and rank was attached to specific positions rather than to the persons who filled the positions, employees were required to transfer to different jobs in order to move up the hospital hierarchy. A nurse on a ward could not be promoted within her ward or service unless a position above her opened up. Often, she was forced to abandon the specialty in which she had accumulated years of experience to attain a higher rank. For example, Mme. Aloncle, who received a distinguished service medal from the Assistance Publique administration in 1899, had entered the Salpêtrière Hospice in 1849 as a *fille de service* in general services. The following year she was promoted to *suppléante* in the sick wards. Three years later, she attained the rank of *sous-surveillante* by taking a job as director of the linen services at the Hôtel-Dieu. After six years she returned to the Salpêtrière wards where, in 1875, she reached the top rank of *surveillante*.[73] Instability and lack of coherence among the staff of any given institution was thus built into the system, as was the likelihood that the medical divisions would lose their most competent and ambitious nurses.

Doctors and surgeons in the hospitals had long complained about the difficulty of retaining nurses in their services. Since the best nurses were often the first to seek promotions, physicians frequently found themselves in the awkward position of taking active measures to block their ablest assistants' advancement.[74] In response to the demands of the medical corps and pharmacists, the new regulations stipulated that the care-giving nursing staff would be divided into two, rather than six ranks: the *personnel non-gradé*, which would consist of five classes of *infirmières* and *infirmiers*, and the *personnel gradé*, which was to be made up of three classes of *surveillant(e)s*. A nurse could advance through the classes within the grade and receive the corresponding salary increases without transferring out of her position.

To the administrators and doctors who formulated the 1903 regulations, the efficacy of all structural reforms in hospital nursing depended ultimately on the complete feminization of the profession. The 1903 statements on feminization differed little from earlier attestations of women's superior aptitude for the profession, except in one critical respect: for the first time, the administration recommended the creation of a training school only for women with no counterpart for men. The establishment of a full-time, two-year professional nursing school for women at the Salpêtrière Hospice was, without a doubt, the linchpin of the plan to build "an elite corps solely concerned with patient care." Modeled directly on institutions in England and on the midwifery school at Paris's own Maternité Hospital, the new school combined classroom lectures with three- to six-month-long rotations in the different hospital wards where students served as nurses. Members of the medical and pharmaceutical staff held classes on subjects ranging from basic anatomy and physiology to methods for treating various types of patients and conditions, while senior *surveillantes* offered instruction in preparing special foods and beverages and in running the wards.

The institution was attached to the Salpêtrière Hospice, but it occupied its own pavilion that included individual rooms for the students, a dining hall, common area, and library.[75] Unlike the programs offered at the four hospitals, the new Ecole des Infirmières de l'Assistance Publique de Paris required full-time attendance for two years for all qualifying applicants. Upon passage of the requisite theoretical and practical exams, the student nurses would receive a *certificat* and immediately take their places as *infirmières* on the staff of one of the hospitals. Eventually, the administrators predicted, the *certificat* would be required of every nurse employed in a Paris municipal hospital ward.

Organizers hoped that the new two-year school would attract women from a higher social class. Yet the administrators disagreed on exactly which women they were trying to recruit and which strategies would be most likely to retain them. The most extensive and heated discussions surrounded the issue of mandatory residency (the *internat*) for nursing students. Those who favored residency argued that only by living together with other nurses in the institution itself would the newcomers grow accustomed to hospital life. Administrators maintained that the *internat* guaranteed the safety of the young women, and that if left to their own devices in town, they might well use their stipend to feed their families or enhance their *toilette*.[76] Institutional residency also served the more pragmatic goals of obviating the need to allocate money for adequate room and board in town, while granting the institution greater control over the professional and personal lives of its nursing staff. Administrators maintained, in a hopeful analogy, that the *internat* created an environment of strict discipline not unlike that of a boarding school. Such arguments betrayed both a general unease with the notion of employment for women and a mistrust of their capacity to behave as responsible economic actors. Perhaps most significantly, the strong administrative support for residential living revealed a deep-seated attachment to associational models for women's public service. Though administrators consistently avoided allusions to religious life, opponents of required residency did not hesitate to point out the parallels between the *internat* and the cloistered lifestyle of the religious orders, between a celibate staff and a congregation. Historian Jo Burr

Margadant notes a similar invocation of "monastic living" in the establishment of the elite women's teacher training school at Sèvres during the same period.[77]

But the *internat* had potential drawbacks even for those who basically supported the idea. Mandatory residence effectively restricted the student body to single women, and the administrators were by no means in agreement that unmarried women made the best nurses. Assistance Publique Director Mourier argued that the hospitals should actively try to attract married women to the nursing profession. Mandatory residence, he asserted, served to bar from the school "honorable women without money whose husbands hold poorly paid jobs." It also discouraged "unmarried women from good families whose parents do not want them to become industrial laborers or commercial employees, and who would be happy to see [their daughters] embrace an honorable profession on the condition that they not be separated from [their families.]"[78] Did these women not represent the best hope for improving the profession's reputation? Despite the administrators' professed admiration for the English model of nursing reform, they could not risk alienating the married women, who already constituted a sizeable percentage of the existing nursing staff and were among its most stable members.[79]

In the end, the commission granted external residence in specific cases, with the *internat* remaining the rule. But the discussion itself suggested a telling lack of consensus over which women would be the standard-bearers for the new elite profession. Was the new Parisian model nurse to be a single woman or widow, able and willing "to dedicate her life to the relief of misery in all its forms," or was she to be a married woman, perhaps even with children, who sought to put her domestic and maternal abilities to good use while helping to support a family? The failure of administrators, politicians, and doctors to articulate a clear vision of the elite Parisian nurse in their 1903 regulations revealed a major source of conflict about the identity of the modern professional nurse: the split between those who viewed nursing as a woman's career equivalent to primary school teaching, and those who saw it as a form of skilled labor for which women were especially, if not uniquely, qualified.[80]

Of the three major reforms proposed by the regulations, only the new training school represented a significant attempt to enhance the professional reputation of Parisian hospital nurses. (Both the separation between patient care and general services and the feminization of nursing positions remained long-term, not immediate goals.)[81] The Conseil de Surveillance promoted the Ecole des Infirmières de l'Assistance Publique, which opened in October 1907 in the Salpêtrière Hospice, as a bold step in the transformation of the role of the nurse in the hospital. "The trained, respected nurse, conscious of her mission and imbued with a sense of the nobility of her care-giving profession, is called upon to play a decisive role in the hospitals through her much appreciated collaboration with the doctor," one pamphlet announced. Echoing the principles of the 1903 regulations, the founders of the new school announced the birth of "a profession with its own expertise [*technique*], traditions, and moral obligations." In short, the trained hospital nurse was no longer simply a skilled worker, much less a modified domestic servant; she was a true professional.[82]

The ambitious scheme was not without its critics, however. Among its most vociferous detractors, ironically, were reformers in Bordeaux, whose own efforts to institute British-style nursing training programs were reflected in the design of the Parisian school (see Chapter 3). Both Anna Hamilton, director of Bordeaux's private Maison de Santé Protestante, and Paul-Louis Lande, director of the public Ecole de Gardes-malades Hospitalières at the Tondu Hospital, found the Salpêtrière school well-intentioned but sorely deficient. They maintained that the Paris reformers had failed to envision a truly professional nurse, and that, as a result, the new training program would never elevate nursing from the status of mere occupation to profession. Salpêtrière students spent far too much time in the classroom, Lande contended, and far too little time working in the wards, where the real professional training took place. During the short periods of time they did spend in the wards, they did not serve as part of the staff but only as auxiliaries. Moreover, the untrained and incompetent nurses already working on the wards provided a dismal example for students to emulate.[83]

Some of Lande and Hamilton's hostility could easily be attributed to competitiveness or to honest or feigned ignorance.[84] Anna Hamilton never hesitated to ascribe the deficiencies of professional nursing training in France in general to the inordinate amount of public attention given to programs developed in Paris and the comparative neglect of all provincial innovations. In several letters to American nursing leaders, she complained of "what is called 'centralization' . . . which is a kind of feeling prevalent with most people that whatever is done in Paris, *must* be what is right, and that the province is forcibly wrong."[85] As for Lande's criticism, much of it was, at best, a distortion of the actual conditions at the Salpêtrière school. In reality students spent every morning of their first year in the medical, surgical, and maternity wards. Classroom work, much of which consisted of practical demonstrations, took place only in the afternoons. During their second year, the curriculum consisted entirely of rotations in the different services, including pediatrics, dermatology, ophthalmology, psychiatry, and general night duty.

But Hamilton and Lande's fundamental mistrust of the Assistance Publique's commitment to creating a new liberal profession for women was not without foundation. One of the Salpêtrière's curricular innovations was the introduction of a three-month-long period during the first year devoted exclusively to general and domestic services in the hospitals. During that time, students received instruction in cooking, bed-making, cleaning, laundry, and other duties generally reserved for the non-nursing staff and the low-ranking *filles de services*. Within the school itself, the students were required to do all the cooking, cleaning, and washing for the institution and its inhabitants. The school's organizers argued that by performing the various housekeeping duties in their own quarters, the future head-nurses not only saved the administration money but learned valuable management skills. "In order to command and instruct her subordinates," one publicity brochure stated, "the *surveillante* must herself execute the routine duties of the hospital."[86] A clear distinction between nursing and domestic service or housekeeping had yet to take hold in Paris. As one nursing journal observed, "a good nurse must first be a good housekeeper."[87] The reluctance of the Paris school's organizers to separate the nursing profession from traditional feminine domesticity, together with their hesitancy to abandon congregational-style residency requirements, reveal once again the tenacity of traditional models of women's public service.

The Assistance Publique's insistence that the new "elite" students perform domestic work also suggests a pervasive ambivalence about what socio-economic category the new trained nurses occupied. On the one hand, the Paris administrators (like their Bordeaux counterparts) reveled in lavish descriptions of charming yet simple student living quarters reminiscent of boarding schools or middle-class homes. Each student had her own room with running water, radiator, glass-paneled wardrobe, table, easy chair, and rug. Like middle-class homemakers, the young students would take pride in their modest but impeccable "house." "It is their own house that they are maintaining," wrote the director of the Salpêtrière Hospice, "and the sense of whiteness and order that reigns here belongs to them."[88] In their hours of leisure, the young women could relax and amuse themselves in cozy common rooms and libraries designed to promote the kind of esprit de corps associated with respectable boarding schools for young ladies.[89]

The administrators recognized, however, that by training women for leadership positions and by offering them material accommodations long denied to the existing staff, they ran the risk of creating a serious division within the ranks of the hospital nurses. "Will they . . . constitute an aristocracy and 'take control' from the beginning?" Such an eventuality, administration agreed, posed a "serious threat" to an institution whose role it must be to train nurses who would blend with and enhance the existing staff.[90] On the opening day of the school's second year, the president of the Paris Municipal Council declared that the city government had absolutely no intention of "creating an aristocracy within the hospital personnel."[91] The regulations requiring the students to clean, cook, sew, and perform other duties normally assigned to the lower-level personnel were undoubtedly intended, at least in part, as a sign that the graduates of the new school did not constitute an elite class of "lady-nurses" set apart from the general nursing staff. The trained nurse of the future was to be a leader among equals; in the words of Gustave Mesureur, director of Assistance Publique, she should be "a higher-ranking worker," not a professional.[92]

Such reassurances notwithstanding, the graduates of the Salpêtrière school encountered considerable hostility in the wards. During the first year of the school's operation, opposition took the form of petty harassment of the students. In some instances, the women sent into the wards for their practical *stage* were virtually ignored by the existing staff and made to stand idly by; in other cases, the students were put to work performing menial tasks usually reserved for the *filles de service*.[93] Much of the resistance stemmed from very real fears among the *infirmières* and *filles de service* that the new graduates would diminish their own chances for promotion. Many believed that the Salpêtrière nurses would be preferred for the higher ranking positions of *suppléante* and *surveillante*, jobs that were perpetually in short supply. The existing nurses feared that the administration would favor the graduates from the new school over nurses with years of experience but an inferior formal training. One nurse of seven years, who had received her diploma from Bourneville's municipal program two years earlier and had attained the relatively high rank of *première infirmière*, anxiously inquired how the entry of the Salpêtrière graduates into the hospitals would affect her professional future:

> Will I have to try all over again for a hospital nurse's diploma? If the students are highly trained, as they are supposed to be, it will hardly be possible for me to compete with them. I would then have to spend my professional life in a lower rank, or transfer to general services . . . Under these circumstances, don't you think that I would be better off waiting no longer, but leaving the hospital and becoming a private nurse?[94]

The Assistance Publique leadership assured the nurses that several years might well pass before the new program attracted any "educated persons of a higher social status." By that time, present-day nurses could attain the rank of *surveillante*. It would be at least another thirty years before the new school had produced enough graduates to fill all two thousand positions of *infirmière, suppléante*, and *surveillante* in the Paris public hospitals.

Yet the administration could not truthfully state that the perceived threat was not real. The gradual replacement of the existing staff of nurses with an elite, highly trained corps of professionals remained, after all, a central goal of the new reforms. Even the Augustine Sisters of the Hôtel-Dieu recognized that the school portended changes in the profession that might soon deprive them of their positions in the city's last three religiously run hospitals. In the fall of 1903, half a year after the administration announced the creation of the new school, fourteen novices from the congregation enrolled in the municipal training program at the Salpêtrière. The occasion marked the first time in the twenty-five year history of the Paris training programs that members of a religious congregation working in Assistance Publique institutions attended public classes. The Augustine Sisters, the *Petit Journal* noted triumphantly, have "succumbed to the force of progress which obligates all corporate groups to move forward, to initiate new methods, or else be charged with inferiority."[95] Only a legal clause and the relative scarcity of lay *surveillantes* with diplomas assured the sisters their positions in the hospitals. The religious nurses recognized that unless they joined the trend toward formal training for nurses, they would soon lose all claim to competence in the field.

Doctors also expressed reservations about the new nurses. Voicing what had already become a familiar complaint in Lyons and Bordeaux, the physicians maintained that the new trained nurses would be "over-educated" after the two-year program and might encroach on the physician's terrain. Dr. Julien Noir, the tireless promoter of nursing as a working-class occupation, feared that the educated woman "will think she knows everything . . . she will dictate to the doctor the wording of his prescriptions."[96] The administration insisted that the program would not produce dangerous "demi-savantes," nor did it herald the birth of a new medical profession. To the contrary, the acquisition of new skills and knowledge was only part of the training the students would receive. Of equal importance was the students' behavior, their "qualities of gentleness and kindness that are particularly feminine qualities."[97] The *Bulletin professionnel des infirmières et des gardes-malades,* whose articles reflected more often the opinions of the hospitals' doctors than those of the nurses, reminded its audience that nursing remained essentially a vocation, not a profession. Despite the administration's efforts to upgrade the educational and social status of the hospital staff, the model nurse in Paris remained Marguerite Bottard, not Florence Nightingale.[98]

Was there any truth to the claim that, within the hospital nursing staff, the Salpêtrière graduates constituted an elite group with better professional prospects? The virtual absence of individual records or even aggregate statistics of the career paths of these nurses makes it impossible to answer this question definitively. Certainly, the Assistance Publique administrators went out of their way to avoid the appearance of granting the Salpêtrière graduates special status or preferential treatment. They insisted that the new school was to take its place among, not above, Bourneville's programs. The new Ecole des Infirmières issued diplomas identical to those delivered by the older programs, in order not to "accentuate the difference of origin or to inflame sensibilities needlessly." Furthermore, there were no formal educational prerequisites for entry into the Salpêtrière school, a point that drew criticism from the Bordeaux reformers. Applicants simply had to pass an entrance exam verifying completion of a primary school education.[99]

Despite these reassurances, some members of the hospital staff remained unconvinced that the Assistance Publique was not setting up a dual-track system of authority and promotion that favored the newcomers. In 1908, the general service *infirmier* and union organizer Abadie reported to the Fédération des Services de Santé de France et des Colonies (the national association of hospital worker syndicates) that the diplomas issued by the two Paris training systems were by no means of equal value.

The degree awarded by Bourneville's one-year programs afforded its recipients no apparent competitive advantage in gaining promotions or salary increases over employees without degrees. By contrast, Salpêtrière graduates were immediately given the rank and salary that normally came only after at least ten years of experience. As a result, young Salpêtrière graduates had authority over many older and more experienced nurses.[100]

Abadie's hostility to the Salpêtrière students was rooted in part in the militant, male-dominated union's (Syndicat du Personnel Non-Gradé) ongoing campaign to block the feminization of all nursing positions, an issue that will be explored in Chapter 5. He scorned the "feminine or nurses' diploma" (as opposed to Bourneville's *diplome mixte*), pointing out that millions of francs had been spent on a school that accepted only young single women.[101] More generally, the union's dissatisfaction reflected employees' fears that the administration had more or less abandoned Bourneville's project of enhancing the reputation of nursing by raising the skill level of the existing staff. Attendance figures seemed to bear out these fears: the number of practicing *filles de service* and *infirmières* enrolled in the new school dropped from nine in 1907, and eight in 1908, to two or three in the ensuing years.[102]

If the Salpêtrière school failed to attract the existing nursing personnel, it had no trouble drawing in young women from all regions of the country. One newspaper estimated that in the fall of 1908, 600 women wrote for permission to take the school's entrance exam, and 250 actually showed up for the test. Although admission required passing an entrance exam but no proof of formal education, many women arrived in Paris with primary-school level *certificats d'études* (about half the class admitted in 1909), and a growing number had the more advanced *brevet élémentaire* (about one-fifth in 1908, and one-third in 1909).[103] While these figures contrast strikingly with the educational profile of the students enrolled in Bourneville's schools, it is worth noting that in 1909 fully half of the women admitted still had no certificates of formal education whatsoever.

The appeal of the new school extended to almost every region of the country, a testimony to both the dearth of professional opportunities for young women and the appeal of the capital city. Between 1908 and 1911, the institution admitted students from 32 to 46 different departments. The largest concentration of candidates outside the Seine came from the three Breton departments, a trend consistent with the general demographic profile of Parisian hospital employees. The southwestern departments of Lot and the Basses- and Hautes-Pyrenées furnished the second largest group.[104] One can only speculate that it was the prospect of finding employment in Paris itself that attracted these young, single women to the Salpêtrière program rather than to the much closer Tondu school in Bordeaux.

Whether the opening of the Ecole des Infirmières de l'Assistance Publique marked a significant step in the transformation of nursing in Paris from menial occupation to respectable profession is difficult to determine. Fifteen years after the institution opened, the Conseil de Surveillance reported that only 70 out of 370 female nurses in Paris were graduates of the Salpêtrière school. The group further acknowledged that those who had attended the program did not appear to benefit from their training either in terms of salary or professional advancement. The administration had successfully guarded against the creation of an elite institution, but in the process had forfeited an opportunity to transform the nature of the nursing profession in Paris.[105]

Still, in the years before the First World War, the administration's claims for the new nurses were grand indeed. Not only was hospital nursing from now on to be considered a stable and lucrative profession, it was suddenly endowed with great symbolic political value. In the rhetoric of the hospital and welfare administrators of the Assistance Publique, nurses had become the cornerstone of social solidarity. The nursing personnel "constitutes an indispensable cog in the social mechanism," the newspaper Les Nouvelles announced in 1909; "it is the repository of a public mission."[106] With red and blue ribbons pinned to their caps, the "Salpêtriennes" served as the "delegates of the City of Paris" to its own poor and sick. It was only a matter of time, AP Director Gustave Mesureur predicted in 1908, before these women "will have added to French prestige overseas, and thus increase the moral patrimony of the Patrie and the Republic."[107]

The complex character of reform in Paris in the three decades before the First World War reveals the limits of any linear, Whiggish model for tracing the history of nursing. While most doctors, administrators, and politicians agreed on the need for reform, they disagreed on what such reform entailed. The sources of their disagreement lay in the unresolved tensions between the familiar nineteenth-century female social roles of wife, mother, and nun, and the newer models of direct public service without reference to family or congregation. While the most doctrinaire anticlericals remained unequivocally opposed to religious nursing, many others made careful exception for the nursing sisters who, in addition to having years of experience on the job, exhibited the desirable qualities of self-abnegation, deference, and lack of personal ambition. Such characteristics appealed not only to doctors who had a clear professional interest in safeguarding their professional dominance in the hospitals, but also to a wide range of republicans who mistrusted the presence of trained lay women in public institutions. As we shall see even more clearly in the next chapter, such men had little trouble reconciling their republicanism with the continuing presence of religious women in the hospitals. One might even say that female religiosity was far less problematic for them than female independence.

CHAPTER

2

The Nursing Sisters
of Lyons

The anticlericalism of Parisian legislators and physicians produced, over the course of thirty-five troubled years, an entrenched if not uniformly trained corps of lay nurses in the capital city. But reformers recognized that policies overtly driven by hostility to the Church and its congregations could not effect similar changes in the provinces.[1] In fact, the Parisian experience served less as a model than as a warning of the potential disarray that could result from the precipitous laicization of hospital nursing staffs, especially in the more conservative provincial cities and rural areas. Anna Hamilton, the Bordeaux reformer who advocated a secular French nursing corps trained along English lines, cautioned in 1900 that

> those who are truly resolved to reform patient services too often adopt measures that laicize hospitals too quickly . . . replacing the *religieuses* with people even less capable of filling the positions; people without honesty or morals. Such measures not only harm the patients whom one is trying to help, but set back real hospital reform which can only be accomplished by a personnel possessing the undeniable qualities of religious sisters combined with the general instruction and technical knowledge that they are lacking.[2]

Even the most avid proponents of laicization agreed that the secular nurse should display the self-abnegation and charitable motivation associated with the congregational nursing sister. A rigorous practical training could enhance her usefulness, but her selfless devotion to the thankless (and minimally, if at all, remunerative) task of caring for the sick and the poor would have to arise from her divinely, maternally, or socially inspired sense of duty. Somehow, politicians had to find a way to laicize nursing staffs without losing the essential qualities on which the vast majority of reformers believed the vocation was based.

Between the salaried Parisian hospital workers and the religious Sisters of Charity stood the hopeful example of the *hospitalières* of the Hospices Civils of Lyons (HCL).[3] In the Lyons "sisters" national nursing reformers saw the best of two worlds: women who undertook a lifelong commitment to serve the sick and poor under harsh physical conditions and with virtually no monetary compensation, but who remained under the direct authority of a secular administration. Ostensibly motivated by religious beliefs, the sisters attended frequent and regular prayer sessions, but they took no vows, adhered to no monastic rule, and were expressly forbidden to form an autonomous congregation. They answered directly to the General Administrative Council of the HCL.

The Lyons sisters drew high praise from republican government officials as well as the republican press. The director of the Assistance Publique administration in Paris noted with admiration in 1891 that the Lyons hospitals had "realized a true miracle, because they have reconciled that which everywhere appears irreconcilable: absolute administrative independence and the spirit of absolute sacrifice among the personnel."[4] The Paris-based *Petit Journal* in 1902 praised the "ingeniously practical and very felicitous 'concordat' . . . of a lay administration and a religious personnel."[5] Similarly, *La Revue philanthropique,* a journal devoted to the official debate on questions of public and private assistance, remarked in 1907 that "this organization has proved itself and produced excellent results. It offers the advantages of a religious spirit, devotion and obedience, and nonetheless has a lay character."[6]

For those republicans who denied the Church's authority in the hospitals but feared the consequences of nationwide laicization, the Lyons sisters stood as evidence that women's religiously inspired virtue could serve the state's interest in providing for the sick and poor. "The current organization, typical of Lyons . . . is the ideal of laicization," asserted Edmond Pellat, an inspector of charitable establishments for the Ministry of the Interior.[7] The conservative proponents of laicization agreed that as long as the Church was stripped of all direct power over nurses as hospital employees, nursing itself could safely remain within the purview of Christian benevolence.

Above all, it was the sisters' devotional quality that made them the most "practical" answer to the question of who should care for the sick and poor. "We must recognize . . . that it is the religious idea that inspires them and sustains them in their arduous vocation," noted Hermann Sabran, then director of the Lyons Hôtel-Dieu, in 1880.[8] The obedience, assiduousness, devotion, humility, and goodwill that characterized the ideal Lyons *hospitalière* also described the dominant virtues of the *religieuse* proper. Caring for the sick and poor was less a job than a vocation, in which service to society was not merely a means to serving God but equivalent to serving God. Without a sense of Christian duty, the *hospitalières* might seek less grueling, less unpleasant, and above all, less hazardous work outside the antiquated, unhygienic, and disease-ridden hospital buildings. Certainly the widespread absence of belief in an obligation to aid the unfortunate would imperil the administration's policy of paying the nurses only forty francs a year. At no time during his tenure as director of the Hôtel-Dieu, Sabran claimed, had he encountered another nursing corps "capable of rendering the same services under the same conditions."[9] The task of the General Administrative Council (GAC) was to protect the *hospitalières'* particular mix of religious spirit and secular direction, "because it will be the surest means to guarantee the practice of charity and tolerance that must be the complement of the life of sacrifice and devotion of a *hospitalière* sister."[10]

The roots of the unique quasi-religious, quasi-lay character of the Lyons sisters lay in a much vaunted and mythologized four-century-old tradition of recruiting young women into a lifelong commitment to caring for the sick and poor who populated the Hôtel-Dieu. The documented history of the *hospitalières* dates back to 1478, when the city's *échevins* (aldermen) took over the administration of the Hôtel-Dieu from the Church. The *échevins* were succeeded in 1583 by a secular board of rectors, which ran the Hôtel-Dieu and Hospice de la Charité until the creation of the General Administrative Council in 1802.[11] The ranks of *hospitalières* were initially composed largely of girls from a variety of socially low-ranking backgrounds, ranging from repentant young prostitutes to orphans who had grown up in the hospices or other public institution. These young women entered the hospital as servants (often literally) and as caregivers to the institution's impoverished residents. According to hospital archivist Auguste Croze, the earliest history of the sisters of the Hôtel-Dieu was fraught with crime and scandal, including reports of illicit relationships between the women and priests and rampant theft by the administrator "mères."[12]

Until well into the nineteenth century, the Lyons nursing corps also in-

cluded a significant number of religiously inspired nursing brothers, called
frères hospitaliers, who served in the male wards, the pharmacies, and in
various administrative capacities. By 1880, however, their presence in the
wards had declined dramatically, and they were no longer being actively recruited. As a result, the brothers were all but ignored by the administration, the press, and the public. The last *frère hospitalier* disappeared from
the sick wards in 1907.[13]

Like their nineteenth- and twentieth-century successors, the first sisters
took no religious vows and remained free to leave the hospital at will.
Like members of a congregation, however, they wore habits, prayed on a
daily basis, and received no payment for their labor. "They are not and
never will be nuns," declared the hospital rectors in the sixteenth century;
"they are but humble servants."[14] Natalie Davis postulates that resistance
to a professing sisterhood during the seventeenth and eighteenth centuries stemmed from fears that the generally elevated social background of
women entering religious orders would entail higher costs for the hospital.[15] Girls and women recruited into the hospitals from the peasantry and
the servant classes, or chosen from among the impoverished hospital clien-
tele itself, could be housed and fed more cheaply than the daughters of
well-to-do families who still constituted a significant percentage of the female religious communities during the early years of the Catholic Coun-
ter-Reformation.[16]

Over the next two hundred years, the rectors formalized the part-secu-
lar/part-religious character of the *hospitalières*. In 1668 they introduced the
ceremony of the *croisure*, in which the sisters who had served for approximately fifteen years received a silver cross as a symbol of their commitment
to the institution where they worked and to the secular authority that gov-
erned them. Despite numerous attempts in the seventeenth century to
transform the sisters into a regular religious order, the administrators refused to surrender their authority. For about a decade during the Revolution the *hospitalières* were forced to replace their silver crosses with patriotic medals, but their ambiguous religious status spared them the official
banishment suffered by the regular nursing orders.[17]

While the dual character of the Lyons nurses often saved them from
anticlerical censure, it did make them the frequent targets of clerical asper-
sions. In 1814, for example, the Restoration government attempted unsuccessfully to force the replacement of the *hospitalières* with the Filles de la
Charité de Saint Vincent de Paul. Accusing the Lyons nurses of "immoral-

ity" and "irreligion," the critics maintained that the sisters contributed to the deterioration of morals among young and old within the hospital walls.[18] Three decades later the government again broached the subject of bringing in the Filles de la Charité, and once more the motion met with resolute opposition from the hospital administration.[19] As late as 1863, a faction of the hospital administration attempted to staff the new Croix-Rousse hospital with the Filles de la Charité de Saint Vincent de Paul. Again tradition prevailed, and instead, a contingent of sisters from the Hôtel-Dieu was transferred to the new institution. The only HCL institution that was staffed by a nursing order by the beginning of the Third Republic was the Hospice des Vieillards de la Guillotière, which was served by fourteen sisters of the Communauté de Saint-Charles until 1909, when the institution was finally laicized. Even then, the Sisters of Saint-Charles were not replaced, but their tie to the *maison-mère* in Paris was severed and their allegiance to the HCL administration secured.[20]

Safeguarding the quasi-religious/quasi-lay character of the *hospitalières* entailed not only preventing their replacement by the Filles de la Charité, but also blocking any internal attempt by the existing hospital sisters and resident priests to undermine the secular administration's authority. In the early years of the July Monarchy, the GAC passed a number of resolutions reducing the powers of the hospitals' resident chaplains *(aumôniers)*. Rising tension over these measures culminated in a brief but dramatic rebellion in the Hôtel-Dieu that became known as the Affaire Gabriel, after Abbé Gabriel, whose influence within the institution threatened secular control over the sisters. The ensuing dismissal of the Abbé in 1834 incited a rebellion among the *hospitalières* that ended with the forced removal of several sisters from the hospital by the police and fifty grenadiers. Although the Affaire ended with the eviction of Abbé Gabriel and many of his most fervent followers, the incident served as a dramatic reminder that the nurses might take it upon themselves to transfer authority to the Church. The HCL administration could not take the *hospitalières'* allegiance for granted.[21]

In the last decades of the nineteenth century the priests' formal administrative power over the nursing staffs diminished even further, and the threat of a clerical challenge to the Administrative Council waned. Although the priests retained "spiritual authority" over the sisters, newly instated chaplains were made to promise explicitly to support the administration and "to watch scrupulously to preserve the spirit and rule of our communities, to remain always the vigilant guard of the institution."[22] Administrators also warned the *hospitalières* repeatedly that attempts to undermine GAC authority would not be tolerated. "Never try to form a religious congregation among yourselves," GAC member Exupéré Caillemer cautioned the sisters of the Croix-Rousse Hospital in 1893, insisting that they "discard all ideas of submission to any monastic suggestion. Remain always . . . under the direct authority of the Administrative Council."[23]

So powerful was the Administrative Council's concern about the allegiance of its nursing staff that it devised a contract between the nurses and the GAC. Signed during the *croisure* ceremony, the agreement bound the sisters "to care for patients always with the same zeal, promising to conform to the Council's orders in cases where the Council feels it must send [the sisters] to another establishment under its authority." In exchange for formal recognition that the secular directors controlled the internal organization of the hospitals, the administration acknowledged its obligation to supply the sisters with food, clothing, and other "necessary items," "in sickness and in health," for the remainder of their lives.

The document was forceful in its delimitation of the administration's duties and in its clear assertion of authority. The GAC's responsibilities to the sisters were entirely contingent on the nurses' "obedience to the rules and orders of the administration, and in the accomplishment of their duty." If the sisters fell short of their obligations in any way, the administration was entitled to expel the culprits without incurring any penalty, "as if this ceremony had never taken place." The GAC was no doubt well aware that a single woman who had devoted fifteen years of her life to hospital service could not risk sacrificing food, shelter, clothing, and, if she survived to claim it, a secure, if not comfortable, old age.

The contract, though clearly intended to formalize the administration's authority and obligations, was also explicit in its articulation of the nurses' rights. Contradicting its own repeated incantations of the signatories' "life-long commitment" to nurse the sick and poor, the document asserted that the sisters remained free to leave the hospitals at any time for whatever reason and without penalty. The sisters did not hesitate to invoke the contract (or if not the actual document, then the spirit of mutual obligation) for their benefit. The minutes of the hospital administration's meetings include scores of examples of monetary compensation awarded to sisters who were forced, usually by illness or family misfortune, to abandon their work. For example, Soeur Clerc, who left the Hôtel-Dieu for "personal reasons" in 1889, after twenty years of service, asked for and received a one-time payment of 500FF.[24] In 1920, Soeur Rendy was allotted 1,000FF after seventeen years in the wards because she was "completely without resources."[25] The Swiss-born Marie Catherine Merck, a *cheftaine* (head nurse) at the Hôtel-Dieu, asked for financial support from the GAC no fewer than seven times after she was forced to leave the country during the First World War. She was awarded nearly 2,000FF.[26] Nurses with shorter records of service, even some who had not yet received the cross, were frequently granted 200 or 300FF.

In doling out these sums on a purely discretionary basis, the administration revealed its reluctance to interpret its obligations in a strictly legal sense, preferring instead to give the appearance of acting out of generosity and sympathy. This paternalistic approach may well have been a calculated strategy to win the allegiance of the sisters, especially during the war, when volunteer lay nurses flooded hospital wards throughout the country, and recruitment figures for the *hospitalières* failed to meet the HCL's needs. Constantly challenged by anticlerical critics from 1880 on, the GAC understood that if it did not show itself to be utterly devoted to the well-being of its nurses, it could not hope to maintain an institution that depended on the voluntary allegiance of the sisters.

The well-known hazards of hospital work made such assurances doubly important. Hygienic conditions were notoriously bad, especially in the oldest and largest institutions like the Charité and the Hôtel-Dieu. Exposed to a myriad of infectious diseases during their ten- to fourteen-hour work days in the wards, the sisters would then retire to living quarters within the hospital that were scarcely less of a health threat. In 1908, for example, the GAC resolved to transform abandoned wards in the Charité into dormitories for the youngest sisters who, until then, had been sleeping in an old laundry room. The old Charité dorms had been the subject of repeated complaints by medical inspectors, who objected to the tiny windows and skylights that made the quarters unbearably hot and stuffy in the summer, glacial in the winter.[27]

Twenty-four hours a day, six days a week, the *hospitalières* worked, ate, and slept in damp, dark, crowded rooms. The sickest nurses, those deemed incapable of performing their professional duties, either returned to their families or became hospital patients themselves. In an attempt to reduce the incidence of tuberculosis among nurses, the hospital directors frequently sent groups of *hospitalières,* especially from the Hôtel-Dieu,

Charité, and Antiquaille (which specialized in treating victims of venereal and contagious disease) to "take the waters" at seaside houses owned by the larger establishments. Even so, tuberculosis remained the leading cause of death or disability among the nurses in years when no typhoid, smallpox, or other epidemic swept the institutions. Only in 1903 did the GAC finally grant the sisters of the Hôtel-Dieu and Charité fifteen days of annual vacation to give them some relief from their noxious environment. During their vacation time, the sisters were not permitted to sleep in their regular quarters. Those who could, were encouraged to spend their time off with their families, for which they were given a 10FF incentive. Those not able to go home would be sent to a country estate belonging to the HCL.[28]

Despite these measures, illness and death remained the most common reason for a sister to leave the hospitals permanently. Of twenty-six women who entered the Charité in the last decades of the nineteenth century, six cited ill health as their reason for leaving, usually after a year or less of work; eight died while in service, and the rest were listed as leaving "voluntarily," which probably meant illness, illness of a family member, or dissatisfaction with the work. Eleven out of the twenty-six left after a year or less, while four stayed for more than thirty-five years.[29]

Why, given these working conditions, would a young woman choose to devote her life to work in the hospitals? The fact that almost all the young women who entered the Hôtel-Dieu and the Charité as novices came from rural regions of the Rhône and the departments immediately surrounding it suggests that hospital service was a reasonable alternative to domestic work for young women looking for employment in the city. Of those whose father's occupation is known, most were daughters of farmers, although a few came from families that practiced such crafts as blacksmithing, clog-making, and weaving, or were involved in small businesses. Some of the prospective novices arrived with letters of recommendation in hand from their local priests and certificates attesting to the upstanding character of the candidate's almost always impoverished family.

But there are hints that at least some young women saw hospital work not merely as a way to survive city life, but as a means of economic and social advancement. Sixteen-year-old Madeleine Richy, for example, arrived in Lyons in the fall of 1902 and applied to become a *hospitalière* at the Hôtel-Dieu. Six years later, with a second-class midwife's diploma in hand, she left for a vacation in the adjacent Saône-et-Loire department, from which she never returned. Shortly thereafter the Hôtel-Dieu administration received a letter from the now twenty-three-year-old Richy confirming her intention not to return to the hospital. Richy's story would hardly be noteworthy, were it not for several distinctive features. First, the girl was several years younger than most novices, who usually were in their twenties when they entered the hospitals.[30] Second, she left her position voluntarily and in relatively good health, an unusual decision for an *hospitalière* with over two years' experience. Most curious of all is a letter addressed to the Lyons municipal council by Madeleine's father, a farmer, in which he requests information about the whereabouts of his daughter. Sent nearly a year after Madeleine's departure from the Hôtel-Dieu, the letter notes that Richy had lost contact with the girl years earlier.[31]

It is possible that Madeleine was sent to serve in the Hôtel-Dieu, with or without her consent, by parents too poor to support her. But why then did her father wait seven years to inquire into her whereabouts? It seems more plausible that hospital service was Madeleine's own idea, to which her father reluctantly (if at all) agreed. We can only guess what motivated the adolescent to break off all contact with her family and travel alone to the city, or why she left for Loisy in the Saône-et-Loire a year after getting a midwife's diploma that authorized her to practice only within the department of the Rhône.[32] We can be reasonably sure only that from the age of sixteen Madeleine Richy was on her own, that while working she took it upon herself to attend midwifery classes, and a year later decided to move on.

Because *hospitalières,* unlike domestics, could receive formal training while working, a six-year stint in the hospitals might have served a destitute but independent-minded or troubled young woman well. Her material needs provided for and her reputation protected by the convent-like character of the nursing *communauté,* the young *hospitalière* would, upon entering the institution, receive schooling in reading, writing, arithmetic, and often some music and drawing. Later she could take courses in anatomy, physiology, first-aid, antisepsis, and other health-care and hygiene techniques. Paid an annual stipend of just 80FF, out of which she had to furnish her own clothing, the *prétendante* (a title conferred on sisters after one year of service) could scarcely accumulate savings. Her hopes for economic and social betterment could be pinned only on the skills she acquired and the availability of employment. Given the absence of comparable detail on the lives of other *hospitalières,* it is impossible to assess the representative value of Madeleine Richy's story. The intriguing case is certainly unique in one respect: the vast majority of women who earned diplomas from any of the HCL's training programs—indeed, most of the *hospitalières* who stayed longer than two years—remained in service until they could no longer perform their duties. Either their dedication to the care of the sick outweighed other aspirations, or the health hazards and hard labor of life in the wards did not seem so untenable when compared to the risks of being a poor, single, minimally educated young girl in a big city.[33] Few moved on to try their skills elsewhere.

The biography of the wealthy Jeanne Aynard, in contrast to that of Richy, points not to a yearning for social mobility but to a desire to lead a socially useful life. Aynard's story does parallel that of Richy in the strong suggestion that her decision to join the Lyons nursing sisters was motivated in significant part by a desire to escape from her family. Born in 1873 at her family's château in Charnay, northwest of Lyons, Jeanne was the daughter of Edouard Aynard, deputy from the department of the Rhône and Lyons's most prominent member of the conservative republican Progressistes.[34] Aynard built his 24-year-long career in the National Assembly (1889–1913) on impassioned speeches against the anti-congregation legislation of the early century, especially the law separating Church and state, and in support of *enseignement libre* (the preservation of religious schooling).[35] It was undoubtedly Edouard Aynard's prominence that led a clergyman to write Jeanne's biography.[36]

Presented as the hagiography of a suffering girl and saintly woman who abjured her family's wealth to dedicate her life to the poor and sick, Jeanne Aynard's biography strikes us today as the story of a deeply troubled adolescent. Jeanne sought safety, solace, and a sense of purpose in devoting herself to God and assuaging the misfortunes of others. Her biographer, eager to describe the physical manifestations of her spiritual suffering, wrote that Jeanne was a heavy child who was teased by her brothers and father. As a teenager, she stopped eating and began exercising avidly, and by age seventeen was thin and weak. Her personal crisis lasted until 1893, during which time she refused to eat or to attend mass or confession, and was severely depressed. She moved to her uncle's house during that period for unknown reasons, but her recovery was slow. By the spring of 1894, Jeanne was still too weak to walk.

It was during this time that Jeanne decided to devote her life to the sick and poor. She had been exposed to charity work from an early age; her mother would take the child to visit the Hospice in Guillotière, then run by the sisters of Saint-Charles. Jeanne's paternal grandfather and great-grandfather had both served on the GAC, and her two older sisters had taken Red Cross training courses at the Hôtel-Dieu. At the age of 21 or 22 Jeanne decided to join the Petites-Soeurs de l'Assomption, an order of visiting nurses based in Paris, but either family pressure or her own unwillingness to go to Paris for the novitiate caused her to revise her plans. In the fall of 1896, Jeanne joined the Hôtel-Dieu *hospitalières* in Lyons.

Unlike Madeleine Richy, Jeanne Aynard could not possibly have had economic motivations for entering the nursing community. Nor does religious inspiration seem to have figured prominently in her decision, despite her biographer's claims. What emerges from the letters transcribed in the book is Jeanne's desperate desire to leave her family home and make a "complete rupture" with the world. "The easy life of a rich spinster has always horrified me," she wrote. "One can try to engage oneself in good works, but since one is more or less always in this world, one ends up devoting only short moments to that work."[37] For Jeanne, who apparently had no intention of marrying, the only escape from a life of idle self-indulgence was complete immersion in "good works." Jeanne's commitment to nursing was further strengthened by her clear desire to escape from her immediate family, especially her father. Her biographer noted that whenever Aynard visited his daughter at the Hôtel-Dieu, "the words died on her lips and . . . she remained like ice in his presence. She never overcame her childhood terror of him."[38]

If what Jeanne sought was an accepting and supportive surrogate family, she did not find it at the Hôtel-Dieu. Ostracized by the other *hospitalières* probably because of her education and class background, Jeanne interpreted her misery as a spiritual trial. "Dear God," she wrote in her confessional journal in 1905, "if this fellow nurse continues to be unkind to me, use the pain that it causes to humiliate me."[39] Jeanne Aynard died in December 1913 of an infection caused by an accidental wound to her finger. Her funeral, as purposefully modest as was her life work, was attended by workers and *femmes du peuple*.[40]

Jeanne Aynard was a rarity among the *hospitalières*, and her well-documented experience cannot be generalized for the hundreds of other nurses whose backgrounds, marked by different hardships, shielded them from the psychological trials specific to the daughter of a powerful, wealthy, and conservative family. To a young woman like Jeanne Aynard, hospital service represented an escape from an intolerable home situation to a place where emotional and physical suffering at least appeared to serve some purpose. The regimented life of the *hospitalière* may have felt like a measure of freedom to her. But for the vast majority of young women who, like Madeleine Richy, arrived from tiny towns and rural areas in the Rhône and its neighboring departments, hospital service represented a guarantee of food, shelter, clothing, company, and even a modicum of education in the city. For those with a religiously inspired sense of duty to the sick and poor, or those who, like Jeanne Aynard, sought solace in service for other reasons, the hard life of a *hospitalière* followed in a long tradition of suffering, self-denial, and healing the sick as service to God.[41]

Although contemporary accounts often exaggerated the sisters' piety for political purposes, there can be no doubt that religious beliefs played a considerable role in motivating these women to work in the hospitals. The rural areas that served as the principal recruitment grounds for *hospitalières* were bastions of religious fervor,[42] and the daily routine of the *hospitalière* was dictated by a schedule of prayer and chapel attendance that remained unaltered throughout the period under consideration here. Despite the limits on the priests' formal powers within the hospitals, resident clergymen were in far closer contact with the sisters than were the institution's secular administrators. The chaplains, not the hospital directors or bursars, were responsible for accepting and rejecting applicants, maintaining discipline among the sisters, and looking after their welfare.[43] Although quick to draw upon the absence of a mother-superior as evidence of the lay character of the *hospitalières,* the administration did not hesitate to rely on the priests to fulfill the functions of such an authority. But the difference between a resident priest and a mother-superior was crucial: the clergymen were hand-picked by the GAC, whereas a mother-superior would be selected either by the *maison-mère,* or by the sisters themselves. Under the Lyons system, the priests retained power over the daily routine of the sisters, but ultimate control lay in the hands of the administration.

This hierarchy of authority did not, however, stanch the growing stream of criticism directed at the sisters by the public and by the anticlerical press. From 1880 until several years after the passage of the law separating Church and state, the GAC was repeatedly forced to defend the sisters against charges ranging from intolerance and proselytizing to nothing short of seeking to overthrow the republic. The editor-in-chief of one of

Lyons' largest daily newspapers, the Radical-Socialist *Le Progrès*, expressed outrage in 1880 that a brochure attacking Freemasonry was circulating freely among the patients of the Hôtel-Dieu. "The brochures do not disguise their hatred for the Republic and overtly preach a return to the monarchy, that is to say, civil war," he fumed.[44] The special commissioner sent by the prefect to investigate the charge confirmed that the sisters were distributing several brochures that, under cover of attacking Freemasonry, were "directed against the government, the decrees of March 29 [against unauthorized religious orders], and republican institutions." Hôtel-Dieu director Sabran did not deny that the offending brochures had appeared in the hospital wards, but maintained that priests unaffiliated with the Hôtel-Dieu had brought them into the wards. He conceded, however, that the sisters were to blame for promoting the priests' "work of propaganda." By serving as a sort of fifth column for the priests who stood outside the authority of the administration, the sisters were guilty of insubordination as well as antirepublican propaganda.[45]

As the anticlerical fervor in Lyons rose to a fever pitch during the 1880s, complaints about the sisters multiplied in the press. In April 1881, the *Lyon Républicain*, mouthpiece of the Radical-Republicans, reported a "serious incident" at the Hôtel-Dieu. According to the paper, an elderly patient had become "the object of obsession . . . with regard to religious questions" of one of the sisters. The old man had apparently defended himself "too energetically" against the sister's accusation that he had not taken his medicine; the nurse responded by evicting him from the hospital. Desperate at the prospect of expulsion, the patient stabbed himself in what the paper termed an attempted suicide. As a result of the incident, the patient was put in a straitjacket, and only when an intern happened upon him later in the evening were his medical needs attended to.[46]

The *Républicain* focused on the irrationality of the sister's behavior and her illegitimate use of power in the form of religious coercion and willful violation of established hierarchies of authority in the hospital. By describing the patient as a *vieillard* (though subsequent investigation revealed him to be 39), the paper effectively portrayed him as the helpless victim of an "obsessed" woman. The nurse further abused her position of authority by acting on her own (that is, not on the doctor's instructions) when she "accused" the pitiable "old man" of not taking his medicine, and then compounded the offense by punishing him for defending himself. The eviction from the hospital was another blatant violation of the hierarchy of hospital authority, since only *chefs-du-service* had the authority to discharge patients. The final act of negligence merely added cruelty to the crimes of irrationality, religious coercion, abuse of power, and insubordination.[47] The incident disturbed the GAC both for its direct association of the nurses with religious coercion and for the implied charge that the nurses, with their irrational, obscurantist, and tyrannical behavior, in fact ruled the hospitals.[48] Sabran's investigative report defended the nurse on the grounds that she had behaved within the parameters of the physician's instructions. It was the patient, he argued, who had failed to obey the attendant nurses and doctors, and thus had clearly violated the hierarchy of hospital authority.

As the winds of anticlericalism gathered force in Lyons, the GAC president repeatedly warned the hospital directors that they must guarantee the patients' liberty of conscience.[49] The nurses especially must be made to understand that it was they who were responsible for upholding that cardinal republican principle. "We insist that all patients be treated equally," Sabran told the *hospitalières* and *hospitaliers* of the Croix-Rousse Hospital in 1883, "with the same devotion, with the same abnegation, whatever their nationality, their religion, or their belief."[50] But instead of transcending the clerical/anticlerical debate, the *hospitalières* and their administrators found themselves caught in the crossfire of politics.[51] Between 1880 and 1887, a series of anticlerical national laws and municipal resolutions brought the already heated political climate in Lyons close to the boiling point. The local enactment of the national Ferry Laws on the laicization of public schools reduced the number of religious teachers in Lyons by a sixth and put them in the minority by 1886. The early part of the decade also witnessed the prefectorial approval of municipal measures banning public religious processions in Lyons and expelling four male congregations—the Jesuits, Capuchins, Marists, and Dominicans—from their quarters.[52]

Emboldened by these initiatives, the municipal council passed six resolutions, nearly one a year, urging the General Administrative Council to laicize its nursing staff. Although none of the measures produced the desired effect, or even elicited more than a perfunctory response from the GAC, the regularity with which the councilmen proposed the bills and the various forms that the measures took indicates the political importance that the issue had assumed. The failure of the resolutions speaks to the continued, if weakening, effectiveness of the GAC's insulation from local political currents during the 1880s.

In the spring of 1880, shortly after the passage of the first national decrees on non-authorized congregations, the Lyons Municipal Council issued a polite invitation to the GAC to laicize the hospital personnel and, concurrently, to set up a school to train the new lay nurses. The resolution claimed that the religious staff cost the administration far more than would a lay personnel, presumably because the HCL had to provide each sister with room, board, clothing, and health care for her entire life. The bill's sponsor asserted that the sisters forced the patients to attend religious services, which he considered both a waste of time and an affront to their freedom of conscience. "The Administrative Council," he concluded, "has no power over its personnel who only obey the leader of the congregation."[53]

The municipal council's proposal elicited no response from the hospital administration, but less than a year later the council produced a stronger measure. Unlike its precursor, this resolution did not couple laicization with the establishment of a training school for the new personnel. Instead, it cast the replacement of the *hospitalières* as part of a broad assault on clerical political power. In the name of the people of Lyons, the council demanded the suppression of the budget for the city's religious institutions, the transfer of the ecclesiastically administered Bureau de Bienfaisance (welfare office) to the municipal council, and the abolition of all male and female religious orders in Lyons. The entire proposal, including the laicization of the hospitals, was intended to "put an end to the excess of religious proselytism" that pervaded the city's public institutions. The prefectorial council, whose approval was required for all municipal resolutions, promptly struck down the budgetary measures on the grounds that they exceeded the municipal council's authority.[54] The laicization request, however, was transmitted to the GAC, where, as in 1880, the issue died.

When the council took up the matter of laicization three years later, it was again with the professed intent to eliminate religious intolerance and coercion. This time, however, the councilmen shifted their ideological rationale. Taking issue with the GAC's assertion that the foundation of effective nursing lay in its religious inspiration, the resolution's sponsors claimed that the patients' freedom of conscience would only be secure once the nurses understood that morality was independent of religious belief. The measure thus took aim not simply at the intolerance of the sisters themselves, but at the viability of a nursing vocation predicated on religious inspiration.[55]

The 1884 proposal called for a gradual transition to a lay personnel based on a new conception of the professional nurse. The creation of a training school attached to the hospitals and the incremental replacement of the *hospitalières* by qualified lay personnel would, the councilmen maintained, transform nursing into a profession for hardworking and honorable women throughout the region. Nursing in Lyons would now attract a new type of applicant, one who did not have the disadvantages of either the *religieuses* or the regular lay personnel, "for whom this profession is usually a way of making ends meet." Instead, the positions would be filled by "women who, since their youth, have viewed nursing as an honorable way to support themselves or their families; who have found at the hospitals not just theoretical and practical training, but habits of behavior and professional dignity!" The councilmen sought, in essence, to replace the religious vocation with a social and professional commitment inspired simultaneously by economic necessity and womanly emotional sympathy, and reinforced by substantive training.[56]

The Opportunist Mayor Charles Gailleton eagerly supported this new, conciliatory line. The laicization of the female personnel, he warned, would require a long period of transition to ensure a competent replacement personnel. The head nurses must be trained in schools, and the rest in the hospitals. This combination of formal and on-the-job training would instill in the nursing corps "the *sentiment* of professional courage" and obviate the problems of insufficient competence, stability, and dedication that had resulted from the Paris laicization campaign. Stability would be fostered instead by encouraging the personnel to have families of their own and by guaranteeing a pension to each employee.

But several members of the council would not concede that the forces of clericalism in the hospitals could so easily be disarmed. Mixing lay and religious personnel in a single training school, one legislator argued, would inevitably lead to the "perversion" of the lay nurses and the triumph of the "religious spirit." Another concurred that "it is clear that the religious personnel ruins the lay personnel and that after some time the nurses will all be imbued with the same spirit." The "religious spirit," synonymous here with proselytism and intolerance, was seductive, contagious, and contaminating. Innocent young women who came in contact with the *religieuses* would be drawn in, manipulated, and, unbeknownst to them, infected by the noxious *esprit*. The language, recalling both centuries-old condemnations of witches and the contemporary jargon of hygiene, cast the sisters at once as heretics, seductresses, and putrefying agents in the temple of the republican hospital.[57]

In the end the Lyons Municipal Council, split between moderates and radical proponents of laicization, could not agree on a viable plan for secularizing the HCL nursing staffs. The resolution that finally emerged once again simply urged the GAC to laicize the hospital personnel and "invited" them to "take the necessary measures to achieve laicization as quickly as possible."[58] Sabran's only reply was to reaffirm the GAC's complete support for the status quo. "We believe that the current organization cannot be modified without serious consequences for our patients," he declared, "and we believe that liberty of conscience is completely guaranteed in our wards."[59]

In 1887 the municipal council passed its final laicization resolution of the century, this time framing the issue as part of a broader effort to secularize the clerically infested HCL. The council voted without discussion to laicize the nursing staff, eliminate the position of resident priest, and have all religious symbols removed from the hospital wards.[60] Ignoring the first two stipulations, the GAC agreed only to remove all religious symbols except images of Christ and the crucifix.[61] By 1920, however, even this measure had not been enacted in all the institutions.[62] That the GAC decided to preserve the most powerful religious symbols in the wards speaks both to their fundamental support for the Christian foundation of sick care, and to their long-standing investment in the possibility that religious fervor could fruitfully be channeled into and subordinated to secular social goals.

After a relatively quiet half decade—between Pope Leo XIII's call for the *ralliement* of Catholics to the republic and the beginning of the Dreyfus Affair—attacks on the nursing sisters increased once again. The Law of Associations of 1901 and the proposal of national legislation on the separation of Church and state under the new Combes ministry in 1902 emboldened the predominantly anticlerical Lyons populace to articulate its dissatisfaction with the hospital personnel. A few years later, the wave of strikes of 1904–1907, the consolidation of the various socialist factions into a unified party in late April 1905, and the long awaited passage of the law separating Church and state in December 1905 galvanized socialist and anticlerical patients (who occupied the majority of hospital and hospice beds) to file grievances against the sisters.[63]

The letters that arrived at the Hôtel de Ville dealt with a range of familiar issues. Most of the complaints echoed those reported in the press and appear almost formulaic in their repetition of certain themes: the sisters disapproved of those who did not practice Catholicism and exerted pressure on them to reform their ways. One patient wrote in 1905 to "formally accuse" the priest of the Hôtel-Dieu of "using the head sister to force a patient to attend Easter services." The writer also noted that public prayer continued to be held in the hospital twice a day, despite regulations forbidding it.[64] A patient at the Croix-Rousse similarly condemned the continued daily practice of morning and evening prayer sessions, while lodging the more serious complaint that the sisters had taken advantage of a patient's loss of consciousness to call the *curé* against his earlier stated wishes.

Other complaints were more suggestive in their critique of the nurses. One 1901 letter composed by several patients reported that the "soeur-mère" [sister-mother] Pillat, recently returned from sick leave, had dismissed patients from the hospital "for the sole reason that they failed to attend mass." In contrast, Pillat's temporary replacement had been "a mother to us."[65] Similarly, another patient in the same hospital accused the head nurse of negligent, distinctly unmaternal behavior in retaliation for his cooperation in the investigation of a charge of religious coercion. Using language redolent of Christian martyrdom, the patient maintained that the sister had denied him morphine to ease his suffering and water to quench his thirst. Like Sister Pillat, this nurse had allegedly gone so far as to threaten to throw the poor patient out of the hospital/home, an act that represented the mother's ultimate betrayal of the child.[66] Complaints such as these, citing political transgressions in terms of violations of codes of gender roles, found an eager audience in an anticlerical municipal council hungry for evidence that the sisters were a threat to society.

It is impossible to determine to what extent these complaints were politically motivated, and to what extent they were founded on genuine dissatisfaction. Whatever the source of the grievances, by the first decade of the century the administration felt vulnerable enough to public criticism to respond to all the letters that reached the prefectoral level, however biased. "Great animosity permeates the Sainte-Marie ward," wrote a Perron Hospice administrator in 1909. "There are two separate camps: those who attend chapel and those who do not . . . . It is unquestionable that the pious patients receive better treatment than the others. The religious zeal of the head nurse must be moderated, as all the disputes in the ward appear to be the result of her propaganda."[67]

But many of the accusations were clearly contrived or arose from ignorance. For example, one M. Gardette lodged a series of complaints against the maternity department at the Charité Hospital, claiming that Soeur

Martel treated his wife roughly, shaved her pubic area to humiliate her, and then asked her inappropriate questions relating to her condition. The ministering physician explained to the prefect that shaving was a standard procedure to prevent infection, especially the deadly postpartum puerperal fever. Furthermore, the sisters were instructed to ask questions about the father of the newborn and any other children the patient might have borne, as the information was relevant to the health of the mother and child.[68]

Although the administrators generally advised the sisters to ignore those who "cast doubt upon your tolerance and make use of the most trivial complaint to accuse you of persecuting those who do not agree with you on religious issues," they nonetheless perceived the rash of complaints as expressing something more than simple political vengeance.[69] Even long-standing admirers of the sisters now occasionally accused them of intolerance and "odious" unfairness.[70] The GAC was forced to admit that the defusing of clerical/anticlerical political tension after the passage of the 1905 law separating Church and state also meant that the institution could no longer take for granted the uncritical support of conservative citizens and politicians. The extreme right-wing monarchists had all but vanished as a political force, and the staunchly Catholic—but avowedly republican— Progressistes resigned themselves, however begrudgingly, to the separation.[71] Unable now to rely on their old political backers for their survival, the sisters had to stand increasingly on their own professional merits.

Fortunately for the Lyons *hospitalières*, the sisters were shielded from much of this criticism by the GAC's unique financial and administrative independence from the Lyons Municipal Council. From the beginning of the Second Empire to 1920, all twenty-five of the HCL administrators were appointed by the prefect.[72] This arrangement contrasted sharply with other provincial cities where, as a rule, the hospital commission consisted of the town mayor and four, six, or eight others. In most cities, the bare majority of commissioners was chosen by the prefect, the rest by the municipal council.[73] The GAC's close political ties to the prefecture gave the conservative hospital administration valuable protection from attacks on its authority by the anticlerical municipal council. For its part, the prefecture, growing wary of the trend toward decentralization of authority over health care, welcomed an alliance that might slow municipal attempts to seize control of urban hospitals.

The administration's autonomy was enhanced by the HCL's unusual (and much envied) financial self-sufficiency. For sixty years—a period of soaring hospital costs resulting from the introduction of expensive new diagnostic and therapeutic techniques and the rising salaries of the increasingly organized medical profession—the HCL managed to balance its budget by drawing on income from a vast array of rural and urban properties as well as charitable donations, bequests, and legacies.[74] Whereas revenues from French hospital holdings on the whole dropped from 45 percent to 30 percent of receipts between 1847 and 1914, in Lyons properties accounted for about 72 percent from 1820 to 1914, and even increased for the period 1860–1904.[75] For the entire period from 1859 until 1918, when the city finally accepted municipal funds to construct the vast new Grange-Blanche Hospital, the HCL received no financial assistance from the municipal council.[76]

The GAC's fiscal and administrative independence from local government made it all the more dependent on private contributions, however, and thus particularly vulnerable to public opinion. In particular, the terms of many bequests and donations included religious stipulations and sometimes even called for joint administration of the funds in question by the GAC and ecclesiastical authorities.[77] "Donations are becoming rarer because many donors and benefactors fear that the conditions that they want to impose on us will not be executed," lamented GAC President Caillemer in 1909. "The number of bequests attached to the saying of masses is very considerable. . . . If the benefactors believe that we do not take into account their desires, they will give their money to other institutions and we will be even less capable of covering our own expenses."[78]

Many donors tied their donations and bequests specifically to the welfare of the nursing sisters. The *hospitalières* thus often served double financial duty as both a cheap source of labor and a lure for fundraising. In 1901, for example, Mlle. Marie Serve de Taluyers left to the Perron Hospice her entire fortune on the condition that a chapel be built for the nursing sisters of the institution. She also bequeathed her mansion to the hospice to be used as a vacation house for the women. A year later, the widow Mme. Rambaud willed 200,000 francs for the completion of the chapel. She likewise gave her house for the leisure use of the nurses.[79] The GAC feared, not unreasonably, that laicizing the nursing corps would cut off vital sources of income from wealthy, conservative donors.

Should such private donations and the HCL's endowment prove inadequate to meet rising hospital costs in the future, the administration would then be at the mercy of the city's industrial and financial elite, whose allegiances tended to economic liberalism, moderate republicanism, and outspoken anticlericalism. These self-styled Radical Republicans dominated the municipal council from 1880 to 1900 and, in coalition with the more left-leaning Radical-Socialists and Socialists, controlled the city government through the First World War. Thus the administration was eager to demonstrate that the *hospitalières* were not *religieuses* at all, but rather the very ideal of women's public service: paragons of self-sacrificing devotion to the weak, helpless, and unfortunate, for the greater glory of God and the republic. Only by promoting such an image of their nursing staff could the administrators hope to transform support of the hospitals into an act of charity apart from the politics of anticlericalism.

By the turn of the century, the GAC faced another threat to its authority from the rapidly organizing medical profession. In 1892, the national government had passed the Chevandier Law granting doctors virtual autonomy in the regulation of the medical profession. Despite a marked increase in public health legislation and continued efforts by the government to coordinate a national health-care program, the 1892 law was considered a clear victory by organized private physicians.[80] As early as the mid-1880s the GAC grew concerned that its perennial rejection of laicization would compromise popular backing for the HCL's autonomy and began soliciting the local doctors' organization, the Comité Médico-Chirurgical, for support for the sisters. The surgeon (and later Socialist mayor) Victor Augagneur recalled in 1889 that the "well-known liberalism of the majority of the members of the *corps médico-chirurgical* was necessary to protect the *religieux* of the hospitals and to struggle against the more or less factitious current of opinion that was pushing for laicization." The powerful professional organization rejected laicization "in principle, in the interest of the patients," but stressed that they supported Lyons' *religieuses* not out of conviction but solely out of concern for the patients. Its support in no way constituted "unqualified approval" of the current system. On the contrary, a "sizeable minority" deplored the insufficiency of the nurses' technical training and called for the creation of a nursing school to ameliorate the problem.[81] This hardly constituted a ringing endorsement of the *hospitalières*.

The doctors remained especially critical of the administration, which they deemed incompetent to make technical decisions affecting hospital care. Throughout the nineteenth century and well into the twentieth, the Lyons hospital administration was dominated by wealthy men with prominent careers in law or finance. In 1909 seven out of the twenty-four regularly elected council members had legal professions, and five were financial administrators, whereas only four were professors at the medical school. Augagneur asserted in 1889 that the medical corps needed to hold at least half the seats in the administration, if it was to play "the role that it deserved." Any lesser representation would only ensure that "decisions would continue to be made by an incompetent majority." Augagneur proposed a neat division of responsibility by which doctors and surgeons would have full control over "technical" issues, leaving administrative and financial matters to lawyers and businessmen. In 1906, however, doctors still held only three out of twenty-five GAC posts; in 1916 that number was reduced to two.[82]

The struggle between the GAC and the doctors for administrative control over the hospitals often took the form of disputes over the *hospitalières*. In 1912, for example, a doctor at the Hôtel-Dieu protested vehemently when the administration transferred the nurse who assisted him to serve as head of the novitiate. Threatening to take the matter up with the Comité Médico-Chirurgical, the doctor argued that the hospital directors were abusing their power and that no changes among the nurses in his service should be allowed without his approval. The GAC, seizing the opportunity to reassert its authority, upheld the decision of the Hôtel-Dieu director, declaring that the "Administrator-Director of each hospital is . . . sovereign judge of the placement of the *hospitalières*. . . . He alone determines the roles that they must fill in the interest of the institution and of the patients."[83]

Power struggles such as this underscored the medical community's lack of support for the administration's policies. Administrators now grew increasingly anxious to prove that the sisters were not an anachronism in the age of "scientific" hospitals. If the Lyons *hospitalières* were to survive, they had to be shown to be in tune with the times politically, morally, and scientifically. "We recognize that progress is unrelenting," Sabran said to the sisters of the Hôtel-Dieu in 1885. "By accepting resolutely the spirit of the century, one can serve one's country without betraying the religious faith to which one is attached." Only through sound general education and substantive professional training could the sisters and their administrators fend off the charges of incompetence that threatened the reputation of the nursing corps. Without such a program, the Lyons hospitalières would soon appear inferior to lay nurses.[84]

Sabran urged the sisters to take advantage of the classes that the GAC had set up in the various hospitals during the past decade. Similar to the programs offered in Parisian municipal training schools, the Lyons courses taught novices basic reading, writing, and arithmetic skills, as well as the elementary principles and practices of nursing. More experienced *hospitalières* could attend evening classes on a voluntary basis. By the last decade of the century, administrators could boast that all sisters had some elementary instruction.[85]

Although touted regularly by the administration as evidence of the sisters' competence and adaptation to modern standards of schooling, these forays into basic education met only with derision from the Comité Médico-Chirurgical. In 1897 Victor Augagneur wrote that everyone had to admit that the "results [of the program] do not measure up to its claims." The present schools, he asserted, "are but an illusion, the *religieuses* learn only words." Similarly, P. Diday, a municipal councilor who generally applauded the sisters' courage and goodwill (which he attributed to their religiosity), conceded that "one could certainly wish for more" with regard to their instruction.[86] Speaking in the name of the Comité Médico-Chirurgical, Augagneur argued that a training school worthy of that title would have a curriculum devised and taught by doctors and surgeons. Departmental heads would evaluate the students' work and divide the graduates into two groups, one consisting of those capable of working in the sick wards, and the other made up of those whose limited abilities required that they remain in laundry, kitchen, and other general services. The plan was intended to steer the most promising students toward patient care. As things stood now, the best candidates often opted to take the less dangerous and better remunerated general service positions.[87]

Concerned above all to protect the nursing sisters who represented its only tangible power base in the hospitals, the GAC voted in the fall of 1899 to create a nursing school for all "persons who want to devote themselves to the care of the sick, whether in the home or in the hospitals." The purpose of the GAC school, the council members agreed, was to provide "professional training" that would allow graduates to "assist doctors, to execute intelligently their orders and to give enlightened care to patients." The new school was to operate under the exclusive direction of the GAC. This clear assertion of authority served to warn both the municipal council and the

Comité Médico-Chirurgical that the GAC would not tolerate threats to its exclusive relationship with the nursing staff, even in the name of scientific progress. In concert with the national Conseil Supérieur de l'Assistance Publique, which only months before had issued a nation-wide call for the creation of nursing schools, the GAC would usher in the age of modern, enlightened hospital care. In so doing, it would demonstrate to all its critics that the sisters of Lyons embodied the future, not the past, of health care in France.[88]

The GAC stressed that the program accepted anyone interested in the nursing profession without regard to religion, belief, or nationality as long as she was at least eighteen years old and capable of writing, "entirely in [her] own hand," a letter of application. But this ecumenical appeal was tempered by a series of requirements apparently devised to discourage applications from independent or abandoned women who might use the school as a means of survival or social mobility; in short, to prevent an influx of women like Madeleine Richy. Unmarried minors had to secure the written permission of the father or guardian; married women were required to seek the consent of the husband and to produce their marriage certificate. Widows had to furnish a death certificate, while divorced and separated women had to produce legal proof of their status. All applicants were required to provide a birth certificate, proof of vaccination, a certificate of *bonne vie et moeurs* (good life and habits) from the mayor of their home town or the local commissioner of police, and where relevant, a copy of their court record. These elaborate documentation stipulations guaranteed that the new professional school would not be used to circumvent marital or familial obligations, and that the conventional hierarchy of decision-making with regard to women's lives would be fully preserved. A young woman who had deserted or otherwise left her home under irregular circumstances had virtually no chance of finding a place in the school.

Candidates were also obligated to submit copies of all certificates and diplomas already earned, and at the very least, be able to produce a *certificat d'études* verifying that they had completed basic primary education. Recognizing that this last requirement would disqualify the vast majority of sisters already in the HCL institutions and discourage rural applicants who formed the core of recruits, the GAC allowed that as a transitional measure, the first year's students could substitute for the *certificat* proof of five years or more experience in private or hospital nursing. Even these candidates, however, would be required to pass a GAC-administered exam establishing their capacity to follow lessons at the new school.

The proposed curriculum conformed exactly to that put forth earlier that year by the Ministry of the Interior's special commission on the problem of nursing training. In fact, the Paris-issued program had drawn heavily on the suggestions of the three delegates from Lyons, the only provincial city represented on the commission. The final report cited the Lyons program's "perfect adaptation to the art of shaping and perfecting the individuals to suit their craft." The Lyons model stressed "the practical spirit and the professional idea," rather than the concepts of anatomy, physiology, and hygiene that characterized the Parisian schools, and which the commission considered excessively detailed.[89]

The nationally circulated report insisted not only on the inherent value of practical, on-the-floor training, but on the deleterious effects of theoretical knowledge of all but the most cursory sort. Theoretical scientific information was to be conveyed only to the extent that it "furthered practical knowledge and allowed nurses to understand the *why* of instructions given to them." To reverse priorities would be to run the risk of favoring "the intellect or only . . . memory" and of "depriving patients of valuable care."[90] But above all, the commission members wanted to prevent a potentially disastrous destabilization of the medical hierarchy that had only recently solidified in the public hospitals. By stressing practical know-how, training schools would "ensure that the nurses were never tempted to take an initiative that belonged to the doctor. The nurse has a very useful but precisely circumscribed role," the commission elaborated. "She is the assistant of the doctor, whose orders she must follow with passive obedience." The nurse must know only enough to be able to report on the patient's condition to the physician, but never enough to be able to venture a diagnosis. The trained nurse occupied a valuable and very specific place in the hospital as the doctor's assistant, not his replacement. The best way to guarantee that she fulfill her appointed role "is to limit her instruction to those things that concern her."[91]

Eager to mollify the medical corps, the GAC in Lyons agreed wholeheartedly with this formulation. The last thing in the world that the administration wanted was to create a corps of *demi-savantes,* whose excess of classroom knowledge emboldened them to encroach on the terrain of the physicians and discouraged the cultivation of obedience, humility, and sympathy.[92] "We willingly acknowledge that instruction alone does not suffice to create a nurse worthy of her title," Sabran noted. The most important qualities of a nurse remained "obedience to her superiors, gentleness, patience, solicitude for all the sick without exception and without preference." Formal training would not change the essential character of the nurse; it would simply enhance her technical skill, which, at least to the majority of legislators and administrators, remained the lesser part of the profession.[93]

The Lyons school's claim to originality lay in its emphasis on the *stage,* or on-the-floor training, as opposed to the more common method of practical demonstrations in the classroom. Because the *stage* took place entirely in the wards, the Lyons program relegated much of the control over the content of instruction to the hospital doctors. The GAC's blueprint mandated a system of rotation by which all students would serve for four hours a day (8 A.M. to 12 P.M.), six days a week, for two months in each of five medical and surgical services: medicine, gynecology, contagious diseases, dressings, and operations.[94] The doctors' reports from this practical internship would form the principal part of the student's school record and figure prominently in the decision whether or not to award a *certificat d'aptitude professionnelle.* In a reversal of the procedures in the Parisian schools, a student could not even take the written test without first receiving satisfactory marks for her *stage.*

The predominance of medical professionals on the jury that reviewed the students' practical performance, oversaw the final theoretical exam, and awarded the certificates confirms that the administration had largely conceded the substance of nursing training to the doctors. It was the Comité Médico-Chirurgical that selected the surgeon and doctor who would offer the classroom lessons. Although the administration controlled admission to the school, the doctors determined the content and boundaries of the nurses' knowledge and responsibility.[95]

Yet within these bounds, the nurses themselves did retain a degree of authority. Nurses who had graduated from the school conducted much of the actual instruction in the wards. Senior nurses, called *monitrices,* taught through example the practical skills of patient care, therapy, assistance in surgery, food preparation management, and direction of linen services. The HCL sisters enrolled in the school were also required to attend daily drills of the classroom lessons, which were similarly directed by experienced nurses at the various institutions.

Despite its limited scope and duration (the year-long program fell short of the nationally recommended two years), the Lyons school nonetheless carried the distinction of being France's first public, full-time training program for nurses. In contrast to programs in Paris, Montpellier, Toulouse, and many other cities (including Lyons itself), where students attended classes for only a few hours a week after work, the new school at the Charité required attendance seven hours per day, six days a week, for ten months of the year. Lyons' hospital administrators, in agreement with the national Conseil Supérieur de l'Assistance Publique, argued that students in the school must be relieved of all other nursing duties in order to be able to devote all their energy to their training.[96] Augagneur, then mayor of Lyons and himself a surgeon, agreed that "one does not learn this profession . . . by warming oneself during the evening in a room where a professor gives some lectures or leafs through some books."[97] Training was no longer simply a matter of supplementing innate talent or religious calling, or refining skills acquired while working in the wards. The opening of the Lyons school, however modest in ambition, marked the first step in the establishment of a standardized professional curriculum for the nursing profession.

Ostensibly open to all interested women of good character and with basic literacy skills, the Lyons training program (and the national model it so closely resembled) took no official position on the sensitive question of the religious or secular character of the trained nurse. Yet for a variety of practical reasons, the school proved far more attractive to the existing Lyons *hospitalières* or, until the law separating Church and state, to members of regular nursing orders than to lay women looking for respectable work. For the nurses already employed by the HCL, enrolling in the school required little adjustment of life style. The women were still housed and fed by the hospitals and still received no monetary compensation for their work. If anything, the seven-hour school day (only a portion of which was spent in the wards) was less onerous than the twelve- to fourteen-hour work days of the Lyons hospital sisters. Similarly, for members of full-fledged religious congregations who enrolled at the Charité school, attendance required a change of venue but no material sacrifice. The congregations continued to support their members during their year of training, and guaranteed them food, shelter, and work after they received their certificate.

But for lay women with no attachment to the HCL beyond their desire to learn nursing skills, school attendance often meant sacrificing a paying job, leaving small children at home, or at the very least, incurring a year's worth of uncompensated living expenses.[98] Women unattached to the HCL or a congregation bore the additional burden of having to seek work after graduation. Nearly all hospitals in the region were staffed by congregations, and few, if any, lay students were willing to enter the ranks of the HCL sisters. Although the administration noted with pride that the lay students who remained in Lyons had been sent to nurse in private homes on the recommendation of the patients' doctors, there is little evidence of widespread collaboration between doctors and trained lay nurses.[99] The GAC did, upon request, furnish the names and addresses of lay graduates who kept the administration apprised of their whereabouts, but beyond this, the administrators made no effort to assist women whose future lay outside the walls of its institutions. There was no formal registry of graduate nurses, and the GAC received very few requests for their services.[100] The consistently modest numbers of lay students enrolled in the school suggests that a *certificat d'aptitude professionnelle* did not automatically open doors, much less guarantee security.

Given the obstacles faced by the lay students, it is not surprising that up to World War I they never constituted more than about a third of the graduating class and usually far less.[101] Dr. M. Durand noted in 1920 that of the 940 women who had passed through the school since its inception, 59 percent had been *hospitalières;* 22 percent had come from religious congregations; and 19 percent had been lay students.[102] Although the *hospitalières* dominated the school for all but two of the first fourteen years of its existence, in 1903–04 and 1904–05 students from religious congregations flooded the school, furnishing half of each of the expanded 70-member classes. This temporary surge undoubtedly reflected the congregations' desire for official credentials in an increasingly anticlerical political climate. The law of associations of 1901 threatened thousands of congregations with dissolution, and the pending legislation on the separation of Church and state had the potential to lock the religious sisters out of all state-funded institutions. The GAC, eager to display swelling attendance figures and insistent that lay and religious elements could coexist peacefully to the patients' benefit, did not hesitate to expand class sizes to accommodate the self-sufficient religious sisters. Congregational domination of the nursing school, however, was fleeting. By 1905–06, in the wake of the law separating Church and state, their numbers dropped to 14 out 48, and in the following year to 4 out of 44.

The predominance of the existing nursing corps in the new program reflected the GAC's real interest, which lay not in broadening the appeal of nursing as a secular career but in protecting the status of its own *hospitalières*. The nursing corps remained the conservative administration's most powerful claim to authority in the hospitals against encroachments by the Comité Médico-Chirurgical, the Ministry of the Interior, and the municipal council. The GAC was less concerned with the real educational and professional benefits of the new nursing school than with the political mileage to be gained from amassing certificates and diplomas. The annual *croisure* ceremonies habitually opened with a tally of degrees awarded to the nurses present and vows to increase the institutional total in the future.[103] Administrators hoped that the degrees would allay continuing doubts about the adequacy of the sisters' professional training.

This, however, they failed to accomplish. In a scathing indictment of the *hospitalières* and the GAC, the Prefect of the Rhône complained to the Ministry of the Interior's Director of Assistance and Public Hygiene in 1910 that, though conceived with the best of intentions, the Lyons program was a "caricature of a nursing school." The prefect maintained that the school was dominated by the resident clergymen and their clerical lackeys within the GAC, who permitted degrees to be awarded to "women without a primary education."[104] Even the school's instructors acknowledged deficiencies. Dr. Chatin complained that many of the HCL sisters chosen to attend the school were too old and had spent too many years developing bad habits in the wards. On his suggestion, the administration decided that those with more than ten years of service would receive a certificate of honorable service that would excuse them from the school, and by 1911, only those aged thirty or younger with five or fewer years of experience were admitted. Furthermore, the rule requiring proof of a primary education would be strictly enforced.

The new regulations had little effect. The administration, unwilling to accept reduced enrollment figures, liberally granted exceptions to the age and experience limitations. Out of the 39 *hospitalières* enrolled in the school for the 1911–12 school year, 19 were over 30 years of age, and the following year 14 out of 38 were above the regulation age. The wartime burdens of personnel shortages and increases in numbers of patients forced the GAC in 1915 to raise the age ceiling to 35 and the service limit to 10 years to prevent the complete collapse of the school.[105]

The Lyons *hospitalières* remained vulnerable not only to criticism of their professional training, but to charges that they were recruited from among a poor, uneducated, naively religious rural population. The prefect

complained to the Ministry of the Interior that the hospital priests were
now completely in charge of finding nurses for the hospitals. The clergymen enlisted "errant priests" in zealously Catholic villages of the Ardèche,
the Haute-Loire, and the Auvergne, who recruited "the least cultivated
women for service in the hospitals. . . . The first condition demanded of
the nurse . . . is the Catholic faith and not an education or a special nursing
vocation."[106]

Although the vitriolic tone of the prefect's letter stemmed from his desire to reveal the clericalism and incompetence of the most reactionary
members of the GAC,[107] his criticism of the educational backgrounds of
the young women who entered service in Lyons' hospitals could not be
contested. Like its Paris counterpart, the Lyons administration acknowledged that most novices in HCL institutions lacked sufficient formal education. Prospective nursing school students were required to demonstrate
proficiency in reading, writing, arithmetic, and basic professional skills before enrollment, and few women chose to expand their basic education beyond the bare minimum. By 1914 only six percent of the sisters had completed the courses and exams required for the *brevet élémentaire*—a degree
that entitled recipients to teach elementary school—even though the hospitals themselves offered these courses.[108] A 1908 attempt to supplement
the *hospitalière*-instructor's lessons with lectures by professors of the *école
normale* met with widespread apathy from the nurses. In 1916, faced with a
renewed threat to the future of the *hospitalières* in the form of thousands of
middle-class women who were entering the nursing ranks during the war,
the GAC voted to create a rigorous new preparatory school under the auspices of university professors.[109] A few years later, only a few *hospitalières*
remained in the classes. The administrators, it seems, could not have it
both ways: if they were going to stress the practical, apprenticeship character of nursing training and trumpet the evils of too much book learning,
they could not expect the sisters to attend classes for degrees that would
have no ostensible effect on their ability to nurse or their future in the hospitals of Lyons. The *hospitalières'* vulnerable position in the increasingly
crowded nursing field became starkly apparent in 1917, when a government order abolished the old exam for the *certificat d'aptitude* and replaced it with a far more rigorous test. The GAC, fearful that many of the
sisters would not be able to pass, designed its own, less exacting admissions
exam.[110]

The GAC's attempts to shore up the *hospitalières'* educational credentials reflected not simply a public relations problem but, more ominously, a recruitment crisis that was affecting a growing number of HCL institutions. As early as 1899, the director of the Asile Sainte-Eugénie requested permission from the GAC to hire two female day workers (at no more than 2FF per day) on the grounds that the current staff of 32 sisters "is not sufficient to meet the needs of the establishment."[111] In 1905, the director of the Perron Hospice noted that recruitment had "practically ceased." Only one novice had entered the institution in the past year, he complained, while deaths and departures had reduced the number of sisters at the hospice from 100 to 94. In addition, twelve *hospitalières* were sick in the infirmary, and three more were attending the nursing school full time. Desperate for help, the hospice hired a forty-year-old widow to serve during the nights and got permission from the GAC to employ two more night-duty nurses.[112]

Seven years later the problem had spread. As GAC President Caillemer reported in 1912, the number of sisters at the hospital had fallen from 251 to 246 over the previous decade, while the number of retired sisters had grown from 12 to 25. The number of active nurses had been reduced by 18, or 7.5 percent.[113] At La Charité, similarly, the staff of 301 *hospitalières* had declined to 284, although unlike the Hôtel-Dieu, the Charité also experienced a substantial drop in the number of hospital beds. The GAC's and sisters' efforts to recruit *hospitalières* from the countryside, especially among the friends and relatives of the existing nursing staff, could not match the growing demand for personnel. By 1916, the ratio of beds to nurse had increased from 7.7 at the turn of the century to 10.6. Four years after the war there was still only one nurse for an average of ten patients.[114]

The *hospitalières* of Lyons never overcame their recruitment problems but, as an institution, they proved to be sufficiently flexible to survive the great legislative changes of the 1920s. The creation of a state-sanctioned national diploma in 1922 resulted in the expansion of the Lyons nursing school's program from one to two years to meet national requirements. A year later, the hospital administrators created a single novitiate for new nurses in order to provide a more uniform and thorough basic education and training.

But the expanding nursing needs of the hospitals could not be met by the sisters alone, and the GAC found itself resorting to hiring increasing numbers of untrained or minimally trained lay *infirmières* and male *infirmiers*. Finally, in 1934, recruitment reached a crisis point, and several hospital services found themselves without any sisters at all. The GAC responded with the creation of the city's first corps of *infirmières civiles* at the new Hôpital Edouard-Herriot.

Still, the Lyons *hospitalières* survived until well into the second half of the twentieth century and even gained a degree of organizational autonomy. As competition from lay nurses forced the GAC to grant concessions to the sisters, they were officially authorized in 1939 to elect their own Superior, responsible for the internal management of each hospital. Although still bound under the secular administration, the sisters now had their own representative council that could advise the Superior, and the Council of Superiors from all the HCL institutions consulted directly with the Administrative Council.[115]

Throughout the thirty-five year period that has been the focus of this chapter, the *hospitalières* of the Hospices Civils de Lyons withstood nearly constant criticism from the municipal council, the anticlerical and republican press, the organized medical profession, and the citizenry of Lyons. What is remarkable about the Lyons nurses is not that they were the objects of so much disparagement during a political era marked, above all, by landmark laws restricting the role of the Church in public life. Far more telling is the fact that the *hospitalières* survived the onslaughts. With their unambiguous place in the hospital medical hierarchy and their clearly stated subordination to secular authorities, the nursing sisters of Lyons had something to offer everyone: the commitment, obedience, and economy of a religious order, and, potentially, the skill and training of a lay nursing corps. The Lyons *hospitalières* stood as evidence, administrators, physicians, and health care reformers agreed, that women's charitable, pious, and maternal impulses could be reoriented from Church-directed to more secular public service.

The *hospitalières* were held out as a solution to the problem of state-Church conflict within the hospitals, not only by the GAC but also by the anticlerical governments of France in the early twentieth century. By accentuating the self-abnegating, maternal, and charitable aspects of the religious vocation and jettisoning any vestiges of autonomy that a religious congregation or order might retain, the Lyons sisters answered the complaints of all but the most radical proponents of laicization, and their most fanatic opponents. For reformers in Paris, the Lyons sisters seemed to embody the reconciliation of the maternal and religious character of nursing with the secular state's obligation to care for its sick and injured citizens.

The organized medical profession, concerned that the growth of hospitals and the flourishing of public health legislation would compromise private practice, found the religious character of the Lyons sisters congenial to the preservation of a single, physician-dominated hierarchy within the wards. By contrast, a religious order with an independent chain of authority would only threaten the physicians' control over patient care. Doctors could also use the *hospitalières* as tools for extracting concessions from the often intransigent GAC. Aware that the conservative administration viewed the sisters as its stronghold within the hospitals, the doctors backed the administration in their defense of the *hospitalières,* in exchange for considerable control over the training, organization, and deployment of the nurses. The GAC, for its part, used the *hospitalières* to curry favor with the doctors. In crafting this alliance, however fraught with tension, the conservative GAC successfully neutralized attacks by the doggedly anticlerical city government.

The example of Lyons' nurses suggested to its many and various supporters a desirable alternative to the image of a new profession for women with all its attendant threats of masculinization and betrayal of women's pious, maternal instincts. The *hospitalières* were living proof that women's labor that had previously served the interests of the Church and the family could fruitfully be harnessed to the state without disturbing the social order. Government authorities had learned their lesson from the bitter controversies that plagued the laicization of Paris's hospitals for almost forty years: only by honoring long-standing traditions of nursing could authority be secularized without compromising the reputation of the occupation. The government needed a more positive model for French nursing than that provided by the Parisian debacle, and in the Lyons sisters the reformers professed to have seen the future, one based on the seamless joining of religious devotion, maternal sympathy, womanly subservience, and secular, scientific training.

Yet it was the hybrid nature of their status and social identity that limited the viability of the *hospitalières* as a model for the rest of France. Indeed, though touted as the solution to the problem of secularizing nursing, the Lyons sisters found no followers. Stalled between vocation and profession, they survived on the strength of their own history and local reputation, on the formidable financial power of the hospital administration, and on the vested interests of medical and political authorities. The failure of the Lyons sisters to serve as a model for hospital nursing in the country suggests that the persistence of women's public service as an activity mediated by the Church or motivated by religious devotion depended on a political, financial, and cultural context whose time had passed. As religion became increasingly identified with the private, feminine domain, religiously inspired public service and the financial and cultural structures that upheld it became increasingly difficult to sustain. Nursing reformers in other cities seized on the maternal, familial aspects of nursing, rather than its religious lineage, as the vehicle for promoting nursing as a respectable occupation, or even career, for women.

3

The *Gardes-malades* of Bordeaux

"Oh, tell me, Madame, when you could stop to gather flowers
along the road, who led you to and kept you in this desolate asylum that is a hospital?"

—RAYMONDE, "OPEN LETTER TO MME. TÉTIGNAC," *LA
GARDE-MALADE HOSPITALIÈRE*

"This service of the sick transformed into a career . . . will soon
constitute the true medicine of women."

—ANNA-EMILIE HAMILTON, "CONSIDÉRATIONS SUR LES
INFIRMIÈRES DES HÔPITAUX"

When 36-year old Anna-Emilie Hamilton submitted her doctoral thesis, entitled "The Role of Women in the Hospital," to the Medical Faculty at the University of Montpellier in 1900, the president of her committee told her "it was all wrong." Nursing, in the opinion of the "good Catholic" Professor Truc, was not a subject worthy of exegesis for the lofty degree of Medical Doctor from the prestigious and deeply conservative Montpellier Faculty. According to the American nursing leader Lavinia L. Dock, even some of Anna Hamilton's "friends and relations . . . were secretly mortified at her selection of a common and unworthy theme. It was almost like selecting the scrubwoman or the scavengers."[1] But within a week, Hamilton later recalled, Truc had conceded that the 500-page study was not only acceptable but remarkable; he recommended only that she delete "some remarks about nuns and an anecdote about Pope Pius." Hamilton's dissertation easily won the approval of her committee. The sole dissenting voice was that of the clerical Professor Estor, who saw the work as a direct assault on the Catholic nursing orders. A year later it was published in its entirety under the title *Considérations sur les infirmières hospitalières*, and in a condensed version as *Les Gardes-malades: Congréganistes, mercenaires, amateurs, professionnelles*.[2]

Anna Hamilton's thesis marked the opening of a new chapter in the history of nursing in France, one in which reformers would attempt to lift the issue of women's work in the hospitals above the fray of the acrimonious clerical/anticlerical political quarrel that overshadowed all discussions of improvements in nursing recruitment and training. The peculiarly French conflation of nursing reform with hostility to the Church, Hamilton argued, had severely hampered efforts to modernize hospital care along the lines laid out by England's Florence Nightingale almost half a century earlier. In Paris, Hamilton's primary target of criticism, politically charged discussions of laicization had seriously misrepresented the issue of reform. Professional nursing instruction itself had become "practically synonymous with hostility toward the Church," a distortion which served only to discourage the most desirable candidates from entering the field. Reformers, she urged, must actively counter the popular suspicion that the new professional training schools were the "enemy camp" opposed to "the Church and God," and instead promote the programs as the gateway to "a new and useful career for educated women."[3]

Dr. Anna Hamilton presented herself to both the French medical world and the international nursing leadership community as the French heir to Florence Nightingale. Like her predecessor, Hamilton stressed the importance of establishing administratively autonomous nursing schools attached to hospitals that would be run by women. She also insisted upon the centrality of on-the-floor hospital training for students and emphasized hierarchy, hygiene, and order in the wards as crucial elements in the transformation of nursing into a vital part of modern medical care and a respectable, even prestigious, profession for women.

Anna Hamilton's perspective on nursing reform was heavily influenced by her deeply felt connections to what she perceived to be an international community of Protestant women reformers. In one impassioned letter to Lavinia Dock, Hamilton complained about the nursing school set up by the prominent Parisian Social-Catholic Léonie Chaptal. "You cannot understand the *French, jesuitie* (sic) and *parisian* mode of acting," she raged, "for Protestant nations consider *truth* in a quite a different way and will ever be surprised; truth is essential to you, it is a detail in Paris."[4] Throughout her career she maintained a regular correspondence with nursing leaders in the United States and England, and proudly noted the numbers of Protestant foreigners among the staff and students of the Maison de Santé Protestante (MSP), the private hospital and nursing school that she directed from 1901 until 1934. If Hamilton was not motivated by specifically denominational goals, she nonetheless believed that just as the Protestant countries (inspired by that consummate Protestant Florence Nightingale) had led the way in nursing reform worldwide, so too was it the task of Protestants to usher the modern age of nursing into France.

Hamilton's own peripatetic life history undoubtedly contributed both to her sense of herself as part of an international reforming community and to her conviction that French nursing urgently needed to be modernized. Born in Italy in 1864 to a father of Irish descent and the daughter of a retired French officer, Hamilton spent her youth in the south of France among wealthy British vacationers. After her father lost most of his money in a land investment scheme in the mid-1870s, the Hamiltons rented out rooms to English visitors. Anna entered the faculty of medicine at Marseille in 1890 as the school's first female medical student after completing a Protestant education in Geneva and a baccalaureate at Chambéry. Financial difficulties soon forced the young woman to interrupt her studies to take on the directorship of the Children's Dispensary in Marseilles, where she spent fourteen months observing the provision of health care. Hamilton resumed her studies at the renowned faculty of Montpellier, convinced that she would write her thesis on the much-needed reform of French hospital nursing. She spent six weeks in England visiting hospitals, and attended a class at the nursing school in Lyons before arriving in Bordeaux.[5]

The reform agenda Hamilton and her co-reformers drew up contrasts sharply with that of Bourneville in Paris and Sabran in Lyons. Whereas Bourneville and Sabran sought to improve the skills of the existing nursing personnel, Hamilton envisaged a radical restructuring and repopulation of the profession. Along with a handful of reformers, including Bordeaux's mayor, Dr. Paul-Louis Lande, she hoped to redefine the function of the hospital nurse as the doctor's essential collaborator and assistant, thereby boosting the nurse's status from that of domestic or religious servant to bona fide female professional. Rejecting the common claim that English and American models of professional nursing would not take hold in Catholic France, reformers in Bordeaux drew liberally on the experiences of foreign reform efforts, hired foreign-trained leaders, and regularly interacted with the international nursing community in an effort to establish a clear professional identity for the "new nurse."

Unlike their counterparts in Lyons and Paris, Bordeaux reformers made a conscious decision to subordinate the issue of anticlericalism to those of class and gender. Although Hamilton was harshly critical of the religious nursing orders in general, she insisted that her advocacy of the laicization of the nation's hospital nursing staffs stemmed not from anti-Catholic or anticlerical prejudice, but emerged logically from an analysis of deficiencies in the religious nurses' performance. Her critique de-emphasized the religious practices of the sisters and ignored entirely the commonplace charge of proselytizing.[6]

Instead, Hamilton argued that the religious sisters everywhere (except in the special case of Lyons where the *hospitalières* performed all nursing duties) had distanced themselves from direct patient care. "They supervise order and cleanliness in the wards, distribute medication and food to the patients, and direct the ignorant and crude male and female nurses, who perform the real patient care."[7] In practice, she maintained, religious nursing sisters were not nurses at all, but supervisors. Their presence in the hospitals split authority in the wards between a religious mother superior and a secular (male) director and effectively blocked the formation of a single medical hierarchy grounded on universal principles of hygiene and scientific health care.

According to Hamilton's analysis, the Catholic sisterhoods could not supply competent nurses because the criteria for recruitment into religious orders and congregations were fundamentally at odds with the demands of the modern nursing profession. The absence of minimum educational requirements for admission into a nursing order meant that many sisters lacked the background necessary to assimilate new therapeutic techniques and theories of hygiene. Moreover, the Catholic denigration of the body as a mere shell for the immortal soul made it impossible for religious practitioners to understand the principles of modern patient care or modern medicine and hygiene in general. "The value of the exquisite cleanliness of pure air, of the outdoors," she wrote, "cannot be grasped by persons whose rules for living stand in opposition to bodily needs."[8] Like the vehemently anticlerical Bourneville, Hamilton charged that most religious sisters, including the Filles de la Charité de Saint-Vincent de Paul who staffed Bordeaux's central Hôpital Saint-André, were unable to perform their full nursing duties because they were forbidden by the rules of their congregation to view or come in contact with unclothed male bodies, even those of boys or male infants. Nursing entailed direct care of the human body as an end in itself. How then could women who had chosen a life dedicated to spiritual perfection through the subordination of physical existence ever fully comprehend the value of modern nursing care?[9]

The religious sisters, in other words, belonged to an earlier age, one that had been overtaken by scientific progress and a secular code of social solidarity. Their continuing dominance in the wards was evidence that French hospitals remained mired in a prescientific age, even as the nation's researchers were changing the shape of medical science. Hamilton did not paint the *congréganistes* as the agents of antirepublican forces, as did Bourneville and many of his fellow anticlerical supporters of laicization. The nursing sisters were simply a constant and humiliating reminder of France's backwardness, of the country's failure to join its northern neighbors at the forefront of medical modernity. They represented less a national threat than a source of national shame.

Hamilton's new nurses would stand in sharp contrast not only to the religious sisters, but to the lay *infirmières* and *infirmiers* who provided much of the actual patient care in the hospitals. Unlike the sisters and the *infirmières*, the modern nurses would enter the profession with a solid general education and a firm grounding in middle-class morals and behavioral codes. They would view themselves as the essential colleagues and assistants of doctors, trained in the most recent theories and practices of hygiene and therapeutic treatment. Nursing would finally take its rightful place among the other medical professions as an essentially humanitarian occupation, whose principal goal was to cure, as well as comfort, the poor and sick.

Hamilton's vision of the modern nurse was deeply rooted in essentialist notions of women's role and capabilities. Women had a "special aptitude" for hospital work arising from their inherently gentle demeanor and their natural desire to ease suffering. Accordingly, the feminization of all nursing positions was an intrinsic part of Hamilton's effort to raise the public prestige of the profession. "We consider male nurses to be naturally incapable of fulfilling the functions of nurses, the crudity of the majority of male nurses is well known . . . This brutality appears to be completely natural."[10] Only an exclusively female nursing corps could maintain the high moral standards necessary to attract educated and well-to-do young women to the profession. Only women possessed the gentleness of manner, the sympathetic touch that soothed the suffering patient.[11]

Being female, though necessary, was not sufficient qualification for entrance into the new English-style nursing profession. The comparative inferiority of French nursing, Hamilton argued, stemmed from the low social origins of the majority of those directly responsible for patient care.

Women from the "servant class" lacked the basic education necessary to master the principles of hygiene and modern techniques of sick care, and lacked the moral fortitude, the *sang-froid* required to handle the myriad crises that arose daily in the wards. The numerous responsibilities of the nurse could only be fulfilled by women "possessing the intellectual culture that refines and develops the qualities of the heart and the spirit; to surrender such a career to persons without such an education would be to discredit [nursing] to a degree for which no diploma could compensate."[12] The modern nurse must have a solid general education, as well as the manners and organizational skills associated with a middle-class upbringing.

Hamilton urged reformers to heed the warning provided by Paris: in the capital, poor women from Brittany and the Franche-Comté used the hospitals as furnished hotels. Hospital administrators, eager to supplement the city's often insufficient and highly unstable staff, indiscriminately hired anyone who appeared at the institutions' portals. Rather than serve as an alternative to domestic work for ignorant and impoverished migrants, nursing must become a real career alternative for the surplus of educated, single young women *sans fortune* who sought teaching jobs or employment in stores and banks.[13]

In essence, the modern nurse must be capable of running patient-care operations at every level, from the purely maternal tasks of comforting and feeding, to the expert, scientific duties of administering sophisticated therapies. It was the nurse who had to bridge the widening gap between the patient population and the rapidly professionalizing, increasingly elite medical personnel. She must be able to offer to each patient the familial solicitude that he (or she) lacked. She must constantly make allowances for the patient and the doctor, meet the needs of science without hurting the patient's feelings, and promote treatment without unduly compromising administrative interests.[14] The delicate task of the modern nurse was to use her innately feminine skills to balance the emotional, spiritual, and physical needs of the patient with the professional and scientific interests of the doctor, and the financial and authoritative needs of the hospital administration.

Hamilton's controversial work was indisputably the most widely discussed treatise on nursing ever published in France. Reformers from Paris to Lyons, and in the United States, England, and Italy praised the book as the first serious French study of the science and profession of nursing. Lavinia L. Dock wrote in 1907 that at the time it was presented, Hamilton's work "was the only serious, extensive, and adequate history of the kind in existence" and "one of the most important landmarks in the modern history of hospitals and nursing."[15]

But Hamilton's work had its detractors as well as its supporters. Her wholesale adoption of the ideology and practices of the decidedly upper-middle-class English reform movement provoked strong criticism not just from defenders of the nursing sisterhoods, but from French nursing reformers themselves. Most prominent among these critics were Parisian doctors Désiré Bourneville and his colleague, Julien Noir. The two outspoken proponents of hospital laicization took issue with Hamilton's trenchant attack on the Paris training schools and with her overall goal of transforming nursing into a strictly middle-class profession. According to Noir, nurses should be chosen from among "those valiant daughters of the people, who, by the power of their intellect and energy, have presented themselves for instruction." A woman of lower-class origins who had herself experienced hardship would be both more sympathetic to her patients' plight and more effective in administering care.

> Still possessing memories of her difficult childhood, this nurse of plebeian origins would be devoid of haughtiness and disdain. She would better understand the patient for whom she is caring, and, knowing how to speak his language, she could more easily win his trust, and would be more likely to find the path to his bruised heart and defiant soul. . . . Her advice would be more carefully listened to than that of the bourgeoise. One does not have to be a psychologist to recognize that the ear believes the voice it is accustomed to hear.[16]

Moreover, Noir added, whereas the "plebeian" nurse expected to perform menial housekeeping and janitorial services, the middle-class woman would shun mundane chores like cooking and cleaning and the more unpleasant duties of patient care.

For Hamilton, however, the elevation of nursing to professional status was predicated on middle-class disdain for domestic work. She insisted that in order to attract more educated and refined candidates to the nursing profession and simultaneously improve the quality of hospital care, skilled nursing duties had to be separated clearly from domestic work in the wards and general services. One of the most obvious failings of the Parisian nurse-training program was its practice of awarding diplomas to men and women who served as common laborers in the hospitals, but who never provided direct patient care. "To assimilate the personnel in charge of direct patient care to employees of this genre," she maintained, "would only damage the reputation of the diploma." Hamilton attributed the failure to differentiate and prioritize among hospital personnel to the old nursing congregations, which, "having not yet understood that the function of the nurse demands special aptitudes, made the sisters work in the linen room, the kitchen, the cellar, the laundry room, even sometimes in the concierge's box, according to the needs of the particular services."[17] Nursing diplomas must be reserved exclusively for women who, born into a social class that endowed them with certain behavioral and moral codes and allowed them access to education, had decided to embark on a career of caring for the sick by mastering a specific body of knowledge and set of practical skills.

Ironically, despite Hamilton's repeated assertion that nursing would join the ranks of respectable middle-class women's professions, in her vision the new corps of nurses resembled far more closely a religious sisterhood than the teachers or office workers whom she invoked. Her insistence that probationers demonstrate a vocational commitment to nursing followed exactly the dictates of Florence Nightingale, who once described the ideal nursing corps as "a religious nursing order under lay control."[18] Hamilton never specified whether the nurse's vocation should be spiritual in nature, but she, like Nightingale, recognized that only women with a profoundly felt need to devote themselves completely to aiding the unfortunate would agree to leave their comfortable, middle-class homes to spend their lives in hospital wards. She saw no contradiction between her efforts to elevate nursing to the status of profession and her belief that becoming a nurse required more than the mastery of a set of professional skills, however sophisticated. "In order to become a career," Hamilton wrote, "nursing must remain nonetheless a vocation."[19]

Like the religious sisters, Hamilton's nurses would agree to a life of celibacy, sacrificing marriage and family to devote themselves body and soul to caring for the sick and poor. Although Hamilton here again drew on the English nursing model, which had itself emerged directly from a tradition of the Anglican sisterhoods, the French reformer denied the analogy with a religious community and instead likened the new middle-class nurses to medical school students. The modern nurse had to be unmarried and childless because, like the medical student, she had to be free to devote all her energy to her hospital service.[20] Pregnancy and child care were incompatible with hospital work. In her analogy Hamilton failed to mention, however, that upon completion of their training doctors were permitted—indeed expected—to marry. Nurses remained, in a sense, perpetual students serving the poor, the sick, the doctors, and the administrators. Unconsciously reversing the logic of Armand Desprès, defender of the nursing sisters in Paris, Hamilton argued that nurses could not serve simultaneously in the hospital and the home.[21] Unlike Desprès, Hamilton found it perfectly acceptable that lay women forego marriage and family to serve the greater public good.

The new nurse would take a place in the hospital's medical hierarchy that was unambiguously subordinate (though never subservient) to the physician. Echoing the observations of her colleagues in the medical profession, Hamilton asserted that "it is extremely ridiculous for a nurse who possesses neither the knowledge nor the rights nor the sex of the doctor, to try to imitate his way of interacting with the patient and to try to use his language."[22] The modern nurse served under the banner of scientific, medical progress, but performed in a distinct, subordinate, but equally important theater. The art of caring meant "meeting the patient's material needs as well as providing consolation and encouragement." This supremely feminine skill "directly complements the 'art of healing.' Both are guided by the scientific spirit for the greatest good of suffering humanity."[23]

While Hamilton acknowledged the physicians' primacy in the single hierarchy that would shape the modern hospital, she insisted that the interior workings of the hospital constituted an inherently female space. Most important—and most controversial—among her administrative reforms was the requirement that only women could serve as directors in charge of the nursing personnel and the institutions' numerous general services (such as food preparation and laundry). Almost all French hospitals were run by male directors with no medical expertise at all. Basing her notion of the *directrice* on the English "matron," Hamilton argued that only a woman could fairly and effectively manage a predominantly female staff.[24] The journal *La Garde-malade hospitalière,* the official publication of the Bordeaux nursing schools, noted in 1907 that "if men were good judges of feminine controversies, it would not have been necessary to create the Directrice. . . . If one wants to guarantee propriety and morality among the nursing personnel, one must select a woman with these qualities as their leader."[25] Women alone were capable of fully grasping the technical, medical, organizational, emotional, and behavioral dimensions of the nursing profession. Though responsible to the doctor on medical matters and to the city's Hospital Administration Commission on budgetary issues, the *directrice* must retain complete control of every other aspect of the internal working of the institution.

Hamilton's insistence on female directorship was driven both by her personal near-obsession with moral propriety,[26] and by her belief that raising the social status of the profession depended on convincing bourgeois families that the hospital wards were as safe as convents.[27] The hospitals would never attract educated, middle-class candidates to the profession if they retained male leadership over the nursing staffs. "Honorable young girls from good families cannot accept the duties of nursing in establishments directed by men. Between [the nurses] and the masculine authority, there must be a maternal and competent woman."[28] The interior of the hospital was to become a female space where men entered only as visitors, distant authority figures, or patients. Doctors would make their rounds once a day and administrators would hand down rules and regulations, but it was the nurses who would transform the wards into surrogate homes for the sick and real homes for the homeless. In other words, the hospital ward was to become a cross between those two sanctuaries of feminine virtue: the convent and the middle-class household.[29]

In attempting to reform French nursing along the lines established in England and the United States, Hamilton and her colleagues faced formidable political and cultural obstacles. The nurses of Bordeaux found themselves combating clerical forces that sought to preserve the field as the province of the Church, anticlerical politicians who hoped to use the new nurses as agents of laicization, and doctors who blanched at the prospect of divided authority (or, worse, professional competition) within the hospital. Convinced that the improvement in the quality of care offered in French hospitals required women's innate and acquired skills, the reformers sent graduates to organize nursing staffs in dozens of cities across the country in the hope of seeding the Florence Nightingale revolution that had never occurred in France. The fact that they only partially succeeded speaks to the persistence of the multiple identities of the nurse as servant, religious sister, and mother, all roles that the Bordeaux nurses explicitly rejected.

The publication of Hamilton's thesis and her subsequent assumption of the directorship of the private Maison de Santé Protestante of Bordeaux in

1901 coincided crucially with Paul-Louis Lande's tenure as mayor of Bordeaux. Lande, himself a physician and member of the Ministry of the Interior's Conseil Supérieur de l'Assistance Publique, actively pushed for the creation of Bordeaux's first municipal nursing school along the lines established at the MSP.[30] Like Hamilton, Lande attributed the deficiencies of French nursing to the inferior education and social status of its recruits. Both envisioned a new profession for French middle-class women and a new position for women working in the hospitals. No longer caretakers of the chronically incapacitated, a custodial position whose inferior status was conveyed by the title *infirmière*, the nurses would hereafter be called *gardes-malades* to signify their role in bringing the patient back to health.

Hamilton and Lande, doctors themselves, sought to redefine nursing to meet, above all, the needs of the medical profession in its newly empowered position in the hospitals. Together, the doctor and nurse would collaborate for the good of an institution that would be less concerned with comforting the old, poor, and feeble than with curing the sick and injured. The Bordeaux *garde-malade* was to be neither a surrogate mother nor a charity worker; she was to be a trained professional. Through her technical training and the deployment of her refined manner and feminine tenderness of spirit, the *garde-malade* would become the modern doctor's most valued assistant.

The key to reforming the nursing profession lay in the creation of a network of rigorous, full-time, two-year training programs, the prototype for which would be the one established at the Maison de Santé Protestante. When Anna Hamilton assumed the directorship of the Maison, the small, private hospital had already been offering courses in sick-nursing sporadically for seventeen years, but the vast majority of the women who sat in on the lectures had no intention of pursuing careers in hospital nursing. Although some probably sought positions as private duty nurses, most of the students were young mothers eager to learn how better to care for their families.[31]

This was not simply a matter of a lack of student commitment to the nursing profession; the training program itself discouraged its graduates from seeking careers by offering no diploma of its own. Bowing to student pressure, administrators finally began allowing the Red Cross affiliated Société de Secours aux Blessés Militaires (SSBM) to confer degrees in 1887, but that organization forbade holders of its diplomas to receive payment for their services as nurses. Thus students who fulfilled the MSP program's requirements came away either with no record of their accomplishment, or with a degree that barred them from accepting a paid nursing position. In 1890 the MSP severed its relationship with the SSBM on the grounds that the latter organization "was not able to handle future professionals."[32]

The administrators of the Maison rejected the Societé de Secours' philanthropic approach to nursing, but never articulated a clear purpose for the MSP program or its students. To Hamilton, the school's director, Mme. Gross-Droz, embodied much of what was wrong with nursing training in France. In private correspondence, Hamilton noted scornfully that Gross-Droz was "the wife of a liquor and sweetmeats manufacturer," held only an SSBM diploma, and "never was a nurse, only attended lectures herself and then became teacher (sic)." Gross-Droz "never perceived the importance of real hospital training and was extremely shocked when I introduced it."[33]

The school's problems were compounded by the policies of the hospital director, the widow Mme. Momméja, who never hired graduates of the institution's training program to serve as nurses in the MSP. Instead, she relied on Protestant women from the Swiss nursing school La Source, in Lausanne, to staff the wards. As a result, graduates of the MSP school seeking a career in nursing had to strike out on their own. Students also had little if any actual contact with patients in the hospital. Only 60 of the 370 women who attended classes from 1884 to 1890 experienced hospital nursing firsthand, and even they assisted the surgeon in the outpatient clinic only two mornings a week. In 1890, after six years of steadily declining enrollment levels, the program was replaced by a two-year school.[34]

But the new, extended MSP program was scarcely more rigorous than the 1884 version. Once a week students attended theoretical lectures and training sessions in the classroom. After passing a series of written tests and a practical exam that included simulated operations (in which the student had to demonstrate her ability to provide "active, conscientious and enlightened support, of true use to the practitioner"), the graduate received a diploma.[35] Even with the new emphasis on practical training and the incentive of a school-issued diploma, the program still attracted primarily auditors with consistently low levels of education. Gross-Droz noted in 1895 that she often used visual demonstrations in her classes in deference to those "barely literate [women] who constitute approximately one half of the student body."[36] While some graduates undoubtedly pursued a career in nursing, the Maison de Santé's nursing school remained a skills-training program, not a gateway to a profession.

With the appointment of Anna Hamilton to the directorship of the MSP, the school underwent a rapid transformation.[37] As in Lyons, the centerpiece of the revamped school was a mandatory, extensive *stage* in the various services of the hospital. But unlike in Lyons, where the student's day was divided between classroom training and practical experience, the MSP program included only one theoretical class per week. Hamilton felt strongly that theoretical knowledge was best conveyed by practical demonstrations, and that true nursing training took place through apprenticeship. "Courses are necessary, even indispensable," she wrote, "but one cannot forget that they are never more than the complement of the hospital *stage*."[38] The student spent most of her six-day work week in the various services under the supervision of graduate nurses, *cheftaines* (head nurses), and the *directrice*. Day duty required the students' presence from 7:30 A.M. to 8:15 P.M. with 2-1/2 hours off, and the night shift (a mandatory part of training) called for 12 hours (8 P.M. to 8 A.M.) on the floor. Every student who received the new diploma of the "Garde-Malade Hospitalière" was required to complete a *stage* of three months in each of the hospital's eight services, in addition to passing a series of exams.[39]

Over the course of the first decade of the twentieth century, the nursing school of the Maison de Santé Protestante promoted a new identity for the nurse, based on the fundamental connection between the feminization and the professionalization of the field. One of Hamilton's first acts upon joining the MSP was to propose the gradual replacement of the male *infirmiers* who staffed the institution's men's wards with the *gardes-malades* in training at the school.[40] The hospital kept some male employees, along with female servants (who retained the title of *infirmières*), to perform heavy labor and domestic chores, but their position bore no relation to that of the trained nurse. The *gardes-malades* had their own sleeping quarters apart from the *infirmiers* and *infirmières*, and ate in a special dining room along with their superiors, the *cheftaines* and the *directrice*.[41] A nurses' salon was added in 1902, the first of its kind in France, where the women could read and relax during their free time.[42] The MSP *garde-malade* occupied an exclusive, separate female space, which remained as distinct from the wards of the indigent patients, laborers, and servants as from the world of doctors and medical students.

Like their English counterparts, the nurses of the MSP school took their places in a hierarchy that successfully maintained its independence from—while remaining subordinate to—the hospital's physicians. Although doctors filled all four positions on the school's examination board and signed each diploma, the MSP *cheftaines* controlled every aspect of nursing care in the wards and the dispensary, supervising students and graduate nurses alike. "Mistresses of ambulatory schools throughout the day," the journal *La Garde-malade hospitalière* noted in 1910, "they never cease to teach, to train the nurses who, by rotation, fall under their orders. . . . They sow— and the patients reap—the good or the bad, according to how the lesson has been delivered and received."[43] Within a system of credentials controlled by the doctors, the MSP nursing leadership maintained authority over the content of the nurses' training and duties.

In keeping with her belief in the innate femininity of nursing, Hamilton placed a great deal of emphasis on character and behavior, both in selecting students among the school's applicants and in grading their performance during the two-year training period. Qualities that included a well-modulated voice, good manners, patience, kindness, calmness, and docility, which in Lyons were deemed to be the products of a religious vocation or charitable calling, were attributed to a proper feminine upbringing at the MSP. Hamilton therefore insisted that admission into the school required a recommendation not from the mayor or local notable, as was the norm for professional training programs, but from a "lady" familiar with the candidate and who could judge the finer qualities of her character. "Certificates from commissioners of police, mayors and other official personages," Hamilton noted, "are considered as not presenting sufficient guarantees on these intimate questions."[44] Affirmation that a young woman came from a moral, devout, and upstanding family could not, in other words, replace the testimony obtained from an "honorable lady" that the candidate met specific gender and class standards.

Once she entered the school, the nursing student was evaluated every month—by the *cheftaine* of each service and the *directrice*—in fifteen areas, only two of which *(activité* and *capacité)* concerned the nurses' execution of medical or technical skills. Hamilton stressed that the remaining thirteen criteria—punctuality, calmness, docility, reflection, uniform, cleanliness, patience, kindness, coiffure, discipline, conscience, manners, and voice—revealed a woman's true aptitude for the profession. Without decent marks in all these categories, no amount of technical expertise or intelligence could win the student an MSP diploma.[45]

The administrators of the MSP proudly and repeatedly claimed that their Ecole Libre et Gratuite des Gardes-malades was the first in the country to offer complete training for the professional hospital nurse, and that the school contained within it the seeds of national reform of nursing care standards. Years of experience at the MSP school and hospital would enable graduates to take the struggle for reform to hospitals across the country and sustain them in the battles they would inevitably have to fight with doctors, administrators, personnel, and even other nursing students.[46] To an extent, these ambitions were fulfilled. Under Hamilton's directorship, the school attracted students from all over France and from several foreign countries. In 1905, for example, the eighteen women enrolled in classes hailed from ten far-flung departments, as well as Algeria and Holland.[47] Similarly, the seventeen first- and second-year students who attended classes in 1909 came from nine departments, including the Drôme, the Seine, the Charente-Maritime, the Tarn, and one from as far away as the Haut-Rhin. Only three came from Bordeaux's own department, the Gironde.[48]

Most of the nurses who received diplomas from the MSP went on to take positions of authority on the staffs of hospitals outside of Bordeaux. Of fifty students who graduated between 1903 and 1910 for whom at least partial career records survive, eighteen served as *cheftaines* or *directrices* in eleven cities, including Albi (Tarn), Alès (Gard), Amiens (Somme), Béziers (Hérault), Cambrai (Nord), Carpentras (Vaucluse), Issoire (Puy-de-Dôme), Reims (Marne), St.-Quentin (Aisne), and Romans and Valence (Drôme). Eight left the profession for marriage. Of the 119 students who had received a diploma by 1916, only 17 had given up nursing entirely; two of them had died, and 12 had opted for marriage. The vast majority of women who completed their training at the MSP remained committed to professional nursing.[49]

The direct influence of Hamilton's project on national nursing reform was limited both by the small size of the institution and by enrollment restrictions dictated by the school's pedagogy. Because students served simultaneously as the institution's nursing staff, the program could only accept as many applicants as the hospital needed to function, usually about ten a year. Typically, the school received at least five applications for each available slot.[50]

What attracted these women to the Protestant nursing school? It is possible that many simply sought a marketable skill by which they could earn a living. Although several obviously wealthy women enrolled, over seventy percent of the graduates during the first decade received complete or partial scholarships to attend the program.[51] Yet the career paths chosen by the graduates suggest that economic need was only one of several factors motivating the women who attended Hamilton's school in the prewar years.

If the scant records of the individual MSP students reveal anything, it is that many of the young women who attended the school were determined to embark upon rewarding and influential careers. While about thirty percent chose to stay in Bordeaux, either as *cheftaines* at the Maison or in other private institutions, many held a succession of high-ranking positions in cities often hundreds of miles away. The widow Gardiol, for example, received her diploma in June 1906; three months later, she departed for Reims to fill a position as *cheftaine* at the municipal hospital. Within two months, however, she accepted an offer to serve as *directrice* of the Hotel-Dieu in Amiens. Less than half a year later the hospital administration of Amiens was dissolved, and Gardiol moved to her hometown of Cambrai (Nord) to serve as *directrice* of the town's civil hospital.[52]

Mlle. Gachon, who graduated in 1904, had a similarly unsettled early professional life. After spending the relatively long span of four years as the *directrice* of the civil and military hospital in Alès (Gard), Gachon became *directrice* of the children's pavilion in a private sanatorium halfway across the country in the Loir-et-Cher. A year later she entered public service again, this time as *directrice* of the civil and military hospital of Béziers on the Mediterranean. Gachon left Béziers within two years to serve as the director of a sanatorium run by the civil hospices of Montpellier.[53]

The career paths of those who pursued hospital nursing indicate that the MSP *gardes-malades* were willing, perhaps even eager, to move from one end of the country to the other to find a position that suited them. But how many choices did these women actually have? As graduates of the Maison de Santé Protestante, they could only find work in laicized or laicizing hospitals whose administrations agreed to pay the salaries that these nurses commanded (in 1907–08, about 1,200FF for a *directrice;* 600–800 for a *surveillante* or *cheftaine,* in addition to room and board). More importantly, employers had to agree to adopt the organizational principles espoused in Bordeaux.[54] Hamilton refused to send graduates to serve in Carcassonne, for example, because the administrative commission there would not replace the male director with a *directrice.* Despite these limitations, MSP graduates managed to capture an impressive number of top-level nursing jobs, given the small size of the school. By 1910, MSP *gardes-malades* had served as *directrices* in six major municipal hospitals outside Bordeaux.[55]

In contrast to the striking mobility of graduates who pursued hospital service, those who opted for private nursing led more geographically stable lives. Almost forty percent of the seventy-two graduates for whom relatively detailed records exist chose to nurse patients in their homes; the majority of these women never relocated. To be sure, private duty nursing required long-term residence in a community in order to build a reputation among the population. But the prospect of a stable residence in and of itself may have presented a certain appeal. Nearly a third of the women who worked as private nurses started their careers in hospitals, but after years of moving from one institution to another, they left the public sector to take positions in private homes for long periods of time. The widow Bouvard, for example, served as *cheftaine* in the Civil and Military Hospital of Alès, the newly laicized Hospital/Hospice of Albi, and in the clinic of Prompt-Secours in Carpentras before trying her hand at private nursing in Nice. Her sister, Mlle. Nectoux, served as *cheftaine* in Bordeaux's Tondu Hospital, was *directrice* of the Hospital of Issoire and of the Civil and Military Hospital of Albi, and then moved to Aix-les-Bain to seek a private position.[56] Clearly, not all graduates were willing to serve as missionaries for the Bordeaux model of professional nursing by accepting a leadership position in an unreformed or reforming hospital. For those who sought instead a stable, respectable means of making a living, home-nursing was an attractive alternative.

Much of the credit for the success of the Ecole des Gardes-malades of the MSP belongs to Hamilton herself. During her thirty-four years as *directrice,* she worked ceaselessly to promote the tiny school both nationally and internationally as the model for nursing training in France. She spoke at or submitted speeches to the International Council of Nursing Conferences of 1907 and 1909, and to the International Conference on Public Assistance and Private Welfare in 1903. From 1905 until her death in 1935, Hamilton corresponded with the most prominent nursing leaders in the United States, describing the tribulations of the Bordeaux-trained nurses who, in their attempt to bring French nursing into the modern era, were forced to do battle with clericalism, political sectarianism, antiprofessionalism, and the entrenched hostility of Paris toward any initiatives emanating from the provinces.

Predictably, not everyone Hamilton encountered admired her ambition and determination. With her strict moral codes and rigid behavioral standards, she struck some of her students as distant and cold, and her refusal to share authority sometimes brought her into conflict with her own colleagues at the Maison de Santé.[57] Still, Hamilton's contribution to the discourse on the changing role of the nurse in the modern hospital was undeniable. An unabashed elitist, she believed the salvation of nursing lay in its firm grounding in middle-class values. She deplored equally the frivolity of the Red Cross society lady who dabbled in heroism and the crudeness of the illiterate servant girl searching for gainful employment. To Hamilton, trained as a doctor, nursing was indeed "la véritable médecine des femmes," requiring both precise and rigorous technical training and refined, feminine behavior.

The first town to take up Anna Hamilton's challenge to reform nursing training along English lines was Bordeaux itself. By October of 1903, when the municipal council finally voted to create a nursing school in the Hôpital Saint-André, the city's Hospital Administration Commission (HAC) was already under considerable pressure from the Ministry of the Interior to set up a school for nurses employed in the hospitals. For months, the mayor (and HAC president) Dr. Paul-Louis Lande and his supporters fought within the HAC to win approval for a two-year program that would be modeled closely on Anna Hamilton's MSP school. The proposed school would admit both lay students and the Filles de la Charité of Saint-Vincent de Paul and of Nevers, who staffed all of Bordeaux's hospitals at the time.

Opposition to the plan was led by the Opportunist former (and future) mayor Alfred Daney, who argued primarily that the city could not afford to support an MSP-style school. But these financial objections masked a deeper ambivalence among many of the commissioners over the future of the religious nursing staff currently running the wards. Although Lande insisted that the new school would be open to "all persons who desire a nursing diploma in order to devote themselves to caring for the sick," many members of the hospital commission and municipal council saw the proposal as a veiled attempt to replace the Sisters of Charity with lay nurses.

As in Lyons, objections to the dismissal of the sisters came not only from conservatives but from staunch republicans, many of whom favored public school laicization. Administrator Lanusse asserted bluntly that he understood the need to secularize education, but believed firmly that "the laicization of the hospitals is not included in the true Republican program." Like many other moderate republicans, he believed that the nursing sisters provided competent service at a bargain price. He saw no contradiction in defending the nursing sisters while opposing the religious teaching orders. Even hospital commissioner Dr. Lauga, one of the principal supporters of Lande's plan, conceded that "the lay element, which is acclimated in the north [Great Britain], would have a much more difficult time . . . in the Latin countries . . . where the presence of religious personnel among the patients is, in some ways, a tradition."[58]

With the HAC at loggerheads over the proposal, Lande enlisted the personal support of the prefect in July 1903.[59] The mere threat of national intervention had its intended effect. Satisfied that experienced religious nurses would be granted second-year status, the commission approved the creation of a municipal nursing school at the Saint-André Hospital on the model of the Maison de Santé Protestante. On October 30, 1903, the municipal council endorsed the vote overwhelmingly.[60]

Much to the disappointment of Lande and his supporters, the decision to create a municipal nursing school marked the beginning, rather than the end, of the struggle to reform nursing in the city's public institutions. Almost immediately, the proposal encountered objections from the clerical press. The most vocal of Bordeaux's conservative journals, *La Nouvelliste,* protested that the entire project was simply an ill-conceived attempt by politicians to force the nursing sisters out of the hospitals. Freely admitting the benefits of formal training, the newspaper argued that the existing supplementary classes for the sisters currently employed at Saint-André met the demands of modern science without incurring the undue expenses of a public, two-year school.

Significantly, the *Nouvelliste*'s chief line of attack was not the superior moral character of the sisters, nor their long and valiant record of courage and devotion to the sick and poor. Instead, the paper protested that the new school would create a completely new hierarchy in the hospital that would challenge the authority not only of the sisters currently in charge of the wards but of the medical students, the midwives, and the doctors. By establishing a separate chain of command whereby students reported to *cheftaines, cheftaines* to the *directrice,* and the *directrice* directly to the hospital administration, the school circumvented the doctor's authority and usurped that of the other medical assistants.

Turning the standard criticism of the religious nurses on its head, the *Nouvelliste* maintained that the sisters' refusal to care for pregnant women and diaper male infants guaranteed that they would not encroach on the responsibilities of the student midwives. The newspaper's editors further contended that in taking over the complete nursing care of several Saint-André wards, the new school personnel—not the religious personnel—held a dangerous degree of autonomy and constituted "a new and perfectly useless cog [in the hospital organization], a continual source of conflict."[61] Unlike the clerical press of Lyons and Paris, the *Nouvelliste* of Bordeaux never claimed that the religious sisters made inherently better nurses; the journal simply maintained that the new nursing school would disrupt current hierarchical chains by redefining the role and responsibilities of the nurse.

The *Nouvelliste*'s most powerful allies in defending the existing organization of hospital personnel and opposing the new "English-style" school were the hospital doctors. The Réunion Médico-Chirurgicale, Bordeaux's powerful doctors' and surgeons' professional association, had long recognized the need for improving the training of hospital nurses, but rejected all aspects of reform that expanded the nurses' autonomy or authority beyond the narrowest limits. The objections centered on the delivery of a diploma and the potential power it held. The majority of Réunion doctors argued that the liberal distribution of "official credentials" could lead to the creation of a new class of "pseudo-doctors" or "sous-officiers de santé" and an increase in the illegal practice of medicine. Given poor people's general preference for charlatans, doctors could not support a proposal that added to the ranks of false practitioners and weakened the bona fide physicians' growing control over the dispensation of medical treatment.[62]

The Réunion members disagreed sharply among themselves over the place of a newly trained nursing staff in the existing hospital hierarchy. One group of doctors proposed dividing the nurses into those who provided direct patient care and assisted the physician in administering medical care, and those who performed general cleaning, maintenance, and domestic labor. The former—which would include all graduates of the new school—would accept orders only from the attending physician, while the latter would serve under the direct orders of the religious nursing sisters, whom the Réunion had no intention of dismissing.[63] In such a schema, the trained *gardes-malades* would be unambiguously subordinated to the doctors.

But the majority of the Réunion maintained that the *gardes-malades*, however well-trained, should remain attached to the religious sisters, not to the physicians. They envisaged a system, modeled directly on the organization of male nurses in military hospitals, by which trained nurses would obey medical orders from the doctors, but answer primarily to the authority of the religious sisters. The sisters would retain control of the daily activity on the wards. Both proposals sought to define a place for the trained lay nurse within the existing organization of the hospital. Viewed as the potential agents of disorder and challengers to the doctors' growing authority, the trained lay nurses were inserted into chains of established authority that confirmed the status both of the medical professionals and of the nursing orders. Lande's project, by contrast, proposed an entirely separate chain of command, with the *garde-malade* responsible neither to the doctor nor to the religious sisters but to the *directrice* and, ultimately, the administration.

When the administration and the municipal council voted in 1903 to accept Lande's proposal without consulting the Réunion, the doctors moved quickly to block what they saw as a major threat to their interests in the hospital.[64] The vociferous Dr. Arnozan, a member of the medical faculty and editor of the *Journal de médecine de Bordeaux*, asserted repeatedly that the new municipal school, like the MSP program, aimed to create an elite corps of nurses whose nominal function was to assist the physicians, but whose organizational principle augured disruption of the status quo. Arnozan even went so far as to argue that granting the *directrice* and her nurses the degree of authority and autonomy stipulated by the new school regulations (and exercised at the MSP as well as abroad) would bring down the republic. Budgetary constraints, he explained, would eventually force the hospital administration to turn to secularized *religieuses* to fill nursing positions. Not long thereafter, "the *directrice* herself will be a secularized nun who one fine day will don again her headdress, and she will no longer be simply the superior of her community, but the superior of the hospital: that is to say, she will have the power to hold both the administration and the doctors in check, as she was once able to do. In this way . . . poorly thought-out reforms will bring about the resurrection of the ancien régime."[65]

Like Dr. Noir in Paris, who denounced Anna Hamilton's "lady nurses" as the products of convents, Arnozan saw the connection between nursing and religious vocation as ineluctable and self-evident. The only way to preserve the secular authority of the doctors and the administrators was, paradoxically, to preserve the authority of the Filles de la Charité, because the sisters' authority derived not from their expertise, however well-trained or experienced they might be, but from the traditional respect accorded women who chose to devote themselves to charitable works. In the existing system, the sisters had no access to administrative or medical power and thus presented no threat to the new medical order in the hospitals.

Although the fervor with which Arnozan expressed his opposition to the school's program exceeded that of his colleagues, there was surprisingly widespread agreement among the Réunion members on the need to protect the religious nursing staff from the discrimination inherent in the project. Experienced nurses, the doctors maintained, would be forced either to enroll in the school, thereby (temporarily at least) giving up their positions of authority, or risk imminent replacement by graduates of the program. When the Réunion met in December to bring about a workable reconciliation between the organized doctors and the mayor, the physicians demanded that Lande "take into account certain rights acquired by intelligent and educated religious sisters that the new [school] rules ignored." After protracted discussions and assurances from the mayor that the experienced sisters would be allowed to enter directly into their second year of training, the group conceded reluctantly that, while flawed, the school represented a step in the right direction. Little would be gained, and much lost, by a refusal to support the project. After all, the Réunion members had been assigned a significant role in teaching, evaluating, and overseeing the students. Their inside influence could be great.[66]

The Bordeaux municipal nursing school opened in January 1904 with a ceremony presided over by its strongest supporters, Mayor Lande and Prefect Lutaud. Gazing out over the assembled crowd that included the entering class of eighteen religious sisters and nine lay students, as well as *cheftaines* from the MSP and from England and a *directrice* from Holland, the mayor reminded the audience of the challenge that lay ahead. The project has been controversial, he admitted, but the school as it was now constituted demonstrated that "the work of charity belongs as much to the lay woman as to the religious sister."[67]

Lande's hopes that the new school would serve as a model for the nation were quickly dashed. Within three months, the HAC received distressing reports that the school had degenerated into chaos. The *directrice*, Mlle. Steffhaan, had failed to organize classes and practical training sessions for the students, who now found themselves performing servants' chores. Dr. Lauga, one of the school's principal proponents, admitted that despite

Steffhaan's unimpeachable credentials, the *directrice* had proved "incapable of being the initiator of an institution whose outline was known, but whose detailed organization must be established by a competent person. . . . She wastes her time with trivial details; she is incapable of setting up a comprehensive plan." Dr. Dupeux, another staunch supporter of the project, added that despite the mayor's constant counsel, Steffhaan had utterly failed to establish her authority, succeeding only in annoying her *cheftaines* by giving orders directly to the students and servants.[68] The school was an unmitigated failure. Five out of the seven HAC administrators in attendance at the meeting on April 8, 1904, voted to replace the *directrice.*

The problems that confronted the school soon reached far beyond the failures of the *directrice* to the fundamental organizing principle of the school and to the collapse of the political coalition that backed it. During his tenure as mayor, Lande had attempted to dispel the political rancor that simmered beneath the thin surface of support for the school by insisting that the program include both religious and lay students. In so doing, he hoped to diffuse the hostility within the HAC and Réunion and appease those on the clerical right who saw the project as an attempt to laicize the Saint-André Hospital.

The fact that the new school was inspired by Hamilton's work at the Maison de Santé Protestante and backed by such prominent Protestants as Gabriel Faure and Lorenz Preller (both of whom sat on the administrative committee of the MSP) only added fuel to the fire of political controversy surrounding the experiment. The reactionary clerical paper *La Croix* claimed that the school was the product of a plot by Protestants and *hommes du bloc* (the center-left republican coalition) to de-christianize France. The *Nouvelliste* accused the school's proponents of attempting to laicize the hospitals of Bordeaux in order to create "openings for the students of the Protestant institutions."[69]

The combination of a hostile political climate and poor organization took its toll. In May 1904, the Socialist minority that had guaranteed Lande's control of the municipal council gave way to a right-wing/conservative/nationalist minority, and the balance of power within the municipal council shifted to the right. The new council promptly appointed the centrist-republican Opportunist Alfred Daney, leader of the opposition to the nursing school within the HAC, to replace Lande as mayor. Supporters of the project justifiably feared for its future under the leadership of a man who had received most of the hard-line royalist and clerical vote.[70] Lande and his backers quickly recognized that the new conservative régime would in all likelihood allow the chaotic situation within the nursing school to escalate in hopes of bringing the whole program to an ignominious end.

Within months after the installation of the new city government, reports reached the prefect of rebellious behavior on the part of the congregational students. "The religious sisters attending the school suddenly tried to elude discipline, to which they only unwillingly submitted," the prefect noted. "They declared themselves wounded in their conscience because they had to obey a Protestant Directrice." At the same time, the lay students felt themselves to be "the objects of insinuations and slanderous comments without finding the protection they needed in the municipal or hospital authorities."[71] Lande, who was immediately appointed by the prefect to replace Daney on the HAC after the latter became mayor, recognized that the only chance of preserving the spirit of rigorous, public, professional nursing training lay in cutting his losses. In August the hospital administration approved Lande's proposal to divide the school into two sections: the Filles de la Charité de Saint-Vincent de Paul and the Filles de la Charité de Nevers would remain in the Saint-André school, while the lay students, *cheftaines,* and *directrice* would take over the nursing responsibilities of the new Tondu Hospital.[72]

Out of the failed Saint-André experiment emerged the secular Ecole de Gardes-malades des Hospices Civils de Bordeaux, which opened at the Tondu Hospital in the fall of 1904. The Tondu school was, in essence, a publicly funded, expanded version of Anna Hamilton's Maison de Santé Protestante. Most of its *cheftaines* and graduate nurses came from the MSP, and the new *directrice*—a former *cheftaine* at the MSP—from England. Despite the collapse of the Protestant-run Saint-André school, Lande continued to assert that the MSP should serve as *the* model for the national reform of the nursing profession.[73]

Local reformers and outside observers alike now began speaking of a "Bordeaux system" of nursing. Admirers predicted that the new *garde-malade*—young, pretty, graceful, intelligent, and well-mannered, dressed in a neat, pale blue uniform—would soon replace the slovenly old nun/servant/nurse draped in heavy black robes who symbolized everything that was wrong with the nation's hospitals. A visitor to Bordeaux's Tondu Hospital in 1906 attributed the success of the nursing school there to the maintenance of strict class divisions among the hospital staff. As soon as the nurses completed their ward duties, he observed, they themselves were attended by servants who served their meals and polished their shoes. The nurses of Tondu, in other words, retained the visible symbols of their middle-class status even in their off-hours. "Look carefully at this abode to understand what the lay nurse can, will, become; she can already be seen in the choice of that vase, the organization of tiny objects on the dressing table, that volume by [Anatole] France, and that sprig of lilac . . ."[74]

In effect, the Tondu nurses presided over a well-ordered bourgeois household complete with furnishings, flowers, photographs, piano, and serving staff. A 1909 promotional booklet issued by the school portrayed the students' living quarters in terms befitting a respectable boarding school for girls. The women are lodged, the brochure noted, in individually decorated, "very pretty little rooms," with "pitch-pine furniture, and glass-paneled armoires." A large common room with a library and piano gave the women a place to gather to talk, sing, or read.[75] In accordance with this new, respectable image, the Bordeaux-trained nurse would oversee the conversion of hospitals across the nation from germ-ridden asylums for the destitute to clean, orderly, spaces that were at once scientific medical institutions and eminently feminine preserves.

Much to their dismay, however, the Tondu and MSP graduates found that their primary national appeal lay less in their skills and refined, middle-class femininity than in their usefulness in promoting secularization. Municipal councils and local hospital administrations from cities all over France requested the services of the *gardes-malades,* hoping thereby to laicize and reform their own institutions. As the agents of radical change, the young women often faced considerable hostility from patients, staff, and the public who supported the religious sisters. Moreover, the self-consciously elite nurses encountered resistance from lay employees who sensed that their own chances for promotion had been jeopardized by the arrival of "imported" nurses. In October 1907, for example, the mayor of Elbeuf in the far northern department of the Seine-Maritime requested a full staff of Tondu graduates to laicize the city's hospital-hospice. The school responded immediately, sending off eight women, six of whom would serve as *cheftaines.*[76] Arriving in the middle of "quite a lively excitement [*effervescence*]" surrounding the eviction of the religious sisters, the young women faced both public hostility and outright antagonism from the existing and newly hired female lay staff. The mayor of Elbeuf noted with chagrin that of the five or six lay assistants who had served under the sisters, only a single male *infirmier* remained; the others had all left.[77]

Female patients and employees were particularly resentful of the Bordeaux nurses, whom they may well have blamed for the abrupt dismissal of the sisters.[78] Given the generally acknowledged higher degree of piety among Catholic women during the Third Republic, it is quite probable that the female patients were more attached to the idea of being cared for by religious sisters than were men patients. The women employees may have objected to taking orders from a lay woman whose only source of authority derived from her superior training and class status. For some, their relationship to the new nurses may have resembled too closely that of servant to mistress. The male personnel, by contrast, probably had little contact with the *gardes-malades,* as men were less likely to be employed in the wards.

The Tondu graduates sent to organize the nursing staff in the new Bodelio Hospital of Lorient, in Brittany, met with an equally chilly reception. In 1904 the municipal hospital administration had decided to open the new institution under the leadership of the Bordeaux nurses, while simultaneously laicizing the city's 300-bed hospice. A year earlier, anticipating the laicization, the administration had set up an eight-month training program for lay nurses, hoping thereby to provide competent personnel for the Tondu graduates.[79] The result fell far short of expectations. The Bordeaux nurses found themselves supervising what they considered to be a severely undertrained corps of predominantly local women with little commitment to the "mission" instilled in the Tondu and MSP students. "The poor nurses appear to have chosen this career as a way to make ends meet," wrote Catherine Elston, *directrice* of the Tondu Hospital school and temporary *directrice* of Bodelio. "They give the impression of store employees who have no taste for their work. . . . One senses that something is missing: training."[80]

Compounding the problem of an insufficiently trained staff were chronic shortages of funds and supplies and relentless criticism from the right-wing press.[81] In 1911 the clerical *Nouvelliste* reprinted Elston's unflattering report on her Lorient experience that had appeared in *La Garde-malade hospitalière,* infuriating the Bodelio administration (as was no doubt the *Nouvelliste* editors' intention). As Hamilton recounted, the Lorient Hospital administration retaliated by vowing to withhold much needed hospital linens.[82] Given the obstacles strewn in the path of the Bordeaux-trained women, it is hardly surprising that between 1905 and 1911 seven successive Tondu nurses served as *directrices* of the Bodelio Hospital.

The attempt by anticlerical hospital administrators (and sometimes mayors) to use the Bordeaux nurses as front-line troops in the battle to laicize hospital nursing staffs brought the new *gardes-malades* considerable national attention. But the Bordeaux nursing leadership was fully aware that this sort of political manipulation presented a potentially lethal threat to the whole reform movement. Elston feared that the inadequacies of the Lorient-trained nurses would fuel the forces that opposed the Système Florence Nightingale. "Lorient made the mistake that so many other places made, and everyone immediately recognized that the faults of the lay nurses are worse than those of the religious sisters."[83] Hamilton also warned repeatedly of the dangers of premature laicization that would "cripple itself by recruiting ignorant and untrained women."[84] The Bordeaux reformers knew that they had to hold themselves aloof, as much as possible, from the purely political struggle for control of the hospitals. They could not simply become agents of laicization but had to retain their carefully cultivated identity as medical pioneers and feminine professionals.

The Bordeaux nurses received little support from the national government in their efforts to separate nursing reform from the laicization agenda of national and local politicians and administrators. When Paul-Louis Lande died in April of 1912, leaving a position vacant on the Hospital Administration Commission, the director of public assistance and hygiene in the Ministry of the Interior immediately wrote to the prefect of the Gironde, Dureault, urging him to appoint a replacement equally "capable of pursuing the work of laicization."[85] Dureault reminded the director that although Lande had believed in the "usefulness of laicization, [he] envisioned its realization only in the relatively distant future."[86] Lande had rejected the substitution of radical laicization for thorough reform and believed that with the proper training, both religious nursing sisters and lay *gardes-malades* could provide adequate care for the sick and poor.

Lande's replacement on the HAC, Charles Cazalet, vowed to continue the work of his predecessor, but the storm clouds of renewed clerical opposition to the school had already massed on the horizon. The appointment of Pierre-Paulin Andrieu, bishop of Marseille, to the archdiocese of Bordeaux in 1909 had marked the end of twenty-five years of relative equanimity within the Bordeaux Catholic community and the beginning of a new era of militant Church opposition to state-sponsored laicization.[87] Adamantly opposed to the republican government, which he accused of Caesarism, Andrieu advocated disobedience to laws that "compromise the most sacred interests of the Church and the family."[88] The reactionary press seized the opportunity created by the death of the popular and respected Dr. Lande to launch a new assault on the Tondu school. "The day after Lande's death," Cazalet wrote in October 1912, the city witnessed a *levée de boucliers* against the school, and demands that the institution close its doors multiplied. "The atmosphere . . . was peculiarly heavy," filled with invective and polemic. "Insignificant incidents were excessively magnified."[89] The editors of *La Garde-malade hospitalière* expressed their anger and bewilderment at the "systematic campaign" directed against the Tondu school. The survival or abandonment of the lay school had become the virtual obsession of the recently appointed hospital administrators, the editors protested, while the school for the religious sisters at the St.-André Hospital continued to function without interference. Furious, the Bordeaux nurses decried the politicization of the nursing profession: "We care for the sick in the hospitals, we are passionately interested in our task in the various social questions that intimately concern our profession, but 'Politics' leaves us completely cold and we can only deplore bitterly that parties out to destroy each other have made us their passive and unwilling prize."[90] But the juggernaut of religious politics prevailed; once again the Tondu nurses were forced to defend their role in the hospitals and prove the legitimacy of their authority.

The school survived the onslaught, but these and other events took their toll. Over the next decade the institution experienced considerable turnover among its leaders. By 1920 Anna Hamilton would describe the Tondu Hospital as "falling to pieces because discipline has become lax and hospital officials have muddled about the choice of undesirable candidates. Girls of the servant class are taken in as pupils and moral behavior is not much thought of."[91] Hamilton's nearly obsessive concern with the "morality" of nursing students aside, the institution's luster faded amid the flurry of activity around public health issues that dominated the immediate postwar period.[92]

Despite widespread acclaim from within the country and abroad, Anna Hamilton's influence in France never approached that of Florence Nightingale in England. By 1914 still only a handful of schools followed Hamilton's model: two in Bordeaux (Hamilton's own Ecole de Gardes-malades Hospitalières at the Maison de Santé Protestante and the municipal school at Tondu), four in Paris (three small public schools and the Ecole des Infirmières de l'Assistance Publique de Paris at the Salpêtrière Hospice), and one each in Béziers (Hérault) and Algeria, both set up and run by Bordeaux graduates. When, in 1923, the Superior Council of Public Assistance and the new Council for the Perfection of Nursing Schools (of which Anna Hamilton was a member) established national standards for nursing training programs along the lines set out by Hamilton, only three of the twenty-eight schools that initially applied for authorization were approved "without reservation": the (renamed) Ecole Florence Nightingale at the Maison de Santé Protestante, the Maison-Ecole d'Infirmières Privées (for private-duty nurses) in Paris, and the Ecole d'Infirmières de l'Hôpital Civil de Reims.[93] Of the three, only the nursing school in Reims was a public institution.

To a large extent, the lack of nationwide enthusiasm for the Bordeaux reform movement can be explained by the impossibility of separating the professionalization of nursing from the politics of anticlericalism in early twentieth-century France. Although the new *gardes-malades* insisted that they would not be used as political tools, the fact remained that to hire a Bordeaux graduate was to establish a secular hierarchy of highly trained women. Thus the new model nurse met with resistance not just from traditionally clerical elements, but also from the nurses' ostensible collaborators—the doctors. The secular *garde-malade* who exercised control over all aspects of ward activity (except for medical diagnosis and the prescription of therapies) presented more of a threat to the doctors' professional ambitions than did a nursing order whose service was understood to be motivated largely by humanitarian and religious charity.

In casting the *garde-malade* as a potential challenger to their authority in the hospitals, the doctors revealed their failure to understand the principles that drove Anna Hamilton's theoretical and practical work. Hamilton's model for the modern nurse was firmly rooted in contemporary views of women's essential character—her natural capacity for sympathy and caring, and her socialized familiarity with cooking, cleaning, bed-making, and other domestic duties. Hamilton and her colleagues went out of their way to define the limits of the nurses' authority as falling within the bounds of a recognizable woman's sphere. The new French nurse was to think of herself as the doctor's assistant and clear subordinate on medical matters, but in her capacity as his closest collaborator, she performed a role as essential to the hospital as the hospital itself was essential to the republic.

The Bordeaux reformers' vision of a professional role for women in the hospitals demanded the reorganization and reassessment of the very function of those institutions. By insisting that women alone could oversee the internal direction of a facility staffed largely by women and devoted to the health and well-being of the population at large, these reformers challenged the authority of both the administrators and the medical profession to define the purpose of state-supported hospitals and to determine how their patients would, in the broadest sense, be treated. One of the editors of *La Garde-malade hospitalière*, calling herself "a modest member of a small group of feminists," explained the formative nature of the *garde-malade*'s work to the large readership of *La Française:* "In our hospital reform movement, it is not our purpose simply to put women at the head of hospitals. We are concerned, above all, to train these women, by compelling them to complete a *stage* of one to two years in a hospital where, under the moral, technical, theoretical, and practical tutelage of women, they themselves will become capable of running houses, households, families and foyers, [all of] which the hospitals must become."[94] The presence of professional middle-class women in the hospitals would shift the institution's primary function from the preservation of social order to the promulgation of masculine medical science and feminine domesticity, albeit in a public setting.

The failure of the Bordeaux reform movement to spawn the revolution in nursing that its leaders had planned can be attributed to a range of factors, both internal and external to Anna Hamilton's original project. The Florence Nightingale System of nursing was a self-consciously feminine professionalizing movement whose measure of success was the growing association of nursing with a specialized body of expertise and a standardized, class-based code of behavior, both hallmarks of established professions. But Hamilton and her fellow reformers in Bordeaux insisted that the future of nursing as a respectable profession lay also in its explicit identification with innate feminine virtues and traditional domestic skills. The *garde-malade* must find her place in the hospital and in the public sphere in general not as a worker or as a *religieuse,* but as a woman.[95]

But in attempting to carve a professional niche for themselves between the ward-servant and the religious sister and between the doctor and the hospital administrator, the *gardes-malades* often found themselves on treacherous ground, without professional authority or public support. As an organized group of women with a clearly articulated allegiance to medical progress and public welfare, the Bordeaux *gardes-malades* presented an unfamiliar threat to established authorities. Deriving their identity from their expertise as well as their sex, these women disturbed the clear alignment of gender, class, and professional hierarchies within the hospital, and in so doing often found themselves less welcome than those potent symbols of reaction, the religious nursing sisters.

4

Class, Gender, and Professional Identity

For nurses in Paris and a few other large metropolitan areas, the first decade of the twentieth century marked the beginning of a long struggle for professional self-definition that would only begin to be resolved after the First World War. This quest assumed a variety of forms which often overlapped and sometimes contradicted one another. The more familiar story—the one that lends itself readily to comparison with the development of nursing in the United States and England—traces the growing emphasis on formal training and credentials that culminated in the establishment of the Salpêtrière Ecole des Infirmières de l'Assistance Publique in Paris and the Tondu Ecole des Gardes-malades Hospitalières in Bordeaux. The creation of these schools suggested a model for professionalization based on the feminization of patient care, as well as such classic professional qualities as restricted entry into the field, mastery of esoteric skills and expertise, and the conscious cultivation of an "esprit de corps" and distinct professional ethos.[1] Reform-minded hospital administrators, politicians, and doctors continually stressed the importance of rigorous training and impeccable moral behavior and heralded the new schools as the "cradle[s] of a new profession for women."[2]

Yet throughout the prewar period, the vast majority of lay hospital nurses in Paris and elsewhere never attended a full-time professional training program. For most nurses, the myth of Florence Nightingale, embedded as it was in strict notions of true middle-class womanhood, had little relevance to their own experience. While professionalizing reformers debated the merits of on-the-ward training and full-time residency at the various nursing schools, hospital employees—the vast majority of whom came from working-class or peasant backgrounds—formed organizations of a variety of political stripes. Between 1892 and 1914, approximately twenty syndicates and unions of hospital nurses, with membership ranging from 6 to 3,500, registered with the Ministry of Labor.[3] In addition, employees established a far larger number of more loosely organized associations and friendly societies. The perspectives and goals of their members, too often lost in the recounting of the history of the "rise of the nursing profession," tell a story that is perhaps more difficult to assemble, but is no less important for its relative obscurity. As Barbara Melosh has argued for the American case, practicing nurses frequently disagreed with their leaders' professionalizing agenda. Most rank-and-file nurses, she notes, "were simply distant from leaders, absorbed in the exigencies and rewards of daily work. It was this shared experience, not the hope of professionalization, that shaped ordinary nurses' aspirations and ideology."[4]

The significance of the various French nurses' associations, however, extends beyond their perennial struggle for the amelioration of their members' material circumstances. Over the course of two decades, the groups served as powerful agents of reform not only of working conditions in the hospitals, but of the public image of nursing itself. The voices of their members constitute a crucial counterpoint to the dominant themes sounded by the professionalizing elite. In an era characterized by official calls for class reconciliation based on paternalist policies and interclass solidarity, nurses and other hospital support staff exposed the contradiction of running public hospitals as if they were part poorhouse and part patriarchal family.[5] The *famille hospitalière* (hospital family) is dead, insisted the most militant of the unions, the Syndicat du Personnel Non-Gradé de l'Assistance Publique de Paris (SPNG). The "secondary staff" should no longer be regarded as domestic servants in the great municipal household of the poor, nor as dependent children subject to the arbitrary authority of superiors.[6] Rather, they should be seen as a special category of workers with specific rights who, as public servants and hospital workers, bore unique and simultaneous responsibilities to their patients, their families, the working class, and the nation.

To a large extent, the emergence of workers' organizations among hospital employees reflected the nationwide intensification of class tensions that marked the dawn of the twentieth century. As historian Judith Stone has pointed out, the first decade of the twentieth century witnessed workers' growing frustration with the Radical Republican government's failure to introduce meaningful labor reforms. The Socialists' withdrawal from the

ruling Bloc de Gauches in 1904 and the establishment of a unified Socialist party (Section Française de l'Internationale Ouvrière, SFIO) in 1905
served to bolster many workers' political opposition to the government.
Nationwide membership in the revolutionary syndicalist CGT (Conféd-
ération Générale du Travail) rose dramatically as a wave of strikes swept
the country. Even the postal workers and teachers, forbidden along with all
civil servants from forming unions, organized illegal strikes in 1906 and
1909.[7] Of the twenty hospital nurses' unions recorded in the Ministry of
Labor's *Annuaire des Syndicats Professionnels* during the two decades before the war, thirteen were established between 1904 and 1909. The fact
that significant numbers of hospital nurses (though certainly not all) identified with the growing discontent of increasing numbers of French workers reveals the limits of the standard professionalizing model for understanding the history of nursing.

The story of the relationship between nursing and organized labor in
France centers, not surprisingly, on the employees of the Assistance
Publique of Paris. In part, this reflects the abundance of sources related to
the activities of nursing organizations in the capital city. Particularly rich
in detail are the police reports on the most militant syndicates' meetings
during the years immediately preceding the war, and the many accounts
from the wealth of Parisian syndicalist and Socialist newspapers. Yet there
are also internal factors that draw the historical spotlight to the capital:
only in Paris did employees of all ranks organize, thus including among
them the men and women most threatened by the Anglo-American model
of simultaneous feminization and professionalization. By contrast, the
membership of the very active Syndicat des Infirmiers et Similaires of the
Hospices Civils de Lyon was limited to those who performed custodial duties or worked in general services. The Lyons syndicate explicitly excluded
the religious *hospitalières*, who held virtually all the hospital nursing positions, and it focused primarily, though not exclusively, on such issues as
wage increases, shorter workdays, sick leave, and vacations, and on efforts
to laicize the hospital nursing staff. Similarly the Syndicat des Employés,
Infirmiers et Infirmières des Hôpitaux et Hospices Civils de Bordeaux
included almost only lower-ranking general staff. Most care-giving and
higher-level positions in the Bordeaux hospitals were occupied either by
congréganistes (at the Saint-André Hospital) or by graduates of the Tondu
nursing school, who were often singled out by the syndicate as the very in-

carnation of the looming threat to its members' livelihood.[8] In Paris, how-ever, where laicization of the hospitals was largely accomplished by the turn of the century, the organized personnel had the chance to shape not only material conditions, but the future of public hospital care.

At first glance, the employees' groups seem to offer a window into at least a part of the working-class nurses' world, a world that is otherwise filtered through the politics and interests of their superiors. But the syndicates and associations, even those whose newspapers or journals are still extant or those whose proceedings have been recorded in police reports, remain highly problematic sources of information about nurses' working lives. Because the largest and most vociferous Parisian groups were organized by rank rather than function, it is unclear whose interests or opinions are being expressed. In other words, the organizations often drew no distinction between nurses (in the sense of those who provided direct patient care) and those who worked in the laundry, the kitchen, or the warehouse. What mattered was not what duties an employee performed, but whether he or she belonged to the upper-tier, supervisory *personnel gradé* or the lower-level *personnel non-gradé*. The Syndicat du Personnel Non-Gradé de l'Assistance Publique de Paris, for example, embraced all salaried employees from *garçon* and *fille de service* to first class *infirmier* or *infirmière*, but excluded all members of the *personnel surveillant*. Some in the SPNG undoubtedly served primarily as *soignant(e)s* (nurses who cared for patients) in the wards, but others worked exclusively in general services or performed strictly custodial duties. Similarly, the enormous Société Amicale des Surveillants et Surveillantes des Hôpitaux et Hospices de l'Assistance Publique à Paris (SASS) included higher-ranking personnel from all divisions within the institutions, but did not distinguish between nurses and general-service workers.

Despite the absence of any rosters identifying the members of the different groups, scattered evidence suggests that both the *personnel soignant* and the *personnel général* participated in collective action. Complaints and requests lodged against the Assistance Publique administration by the SPNG on behalf of its members indicate that adherents performed all manner of functions from simple ward servant to *infirmière soignante*. Of the seven officers sitting on the administrative council of the Parisian Groupement du Personnel Secondaire de l'Assistance Publique in 1900, four were general-service workers and three cared for patients on the wards.[9] Not until after the First World War did hospital nurses who provided sick care on the wards organize as a group apart from their colleagues in the general services.

Does this mean that male and female nurses (*soignant(e)s*) considered themselves first of all to be employees of the hospital administration and of the public welfare system, and only secondarily trained physicians' assistants or health-care professionals? Or does it mean that the nurses who joined the associations and syndicates did so to pursue limited, material goals, and that other important aspects of their professional identity were expressed elsewhere, if at all? At the very least, one must exercise great caution in translating opinions voiced through the organizations into the nurses' beliefs about themselves.

Another telling characteristic of the various employee associations is the general under-representation of women of all ranks and their virtual absence from all organizational leadership positions until well into the First World War. Men dominated the membership of the moderate Societé Amicale des Surveillants et Surveillantes, although women constituted well over half of the Paris AP's supervisory staff when the group was formed in 1904. By December 1913, when the Societé's membership had topped 1,100, only 2 out of 7 of the organization's administrative council members were women.[10] Nationwide, excluding the SPNG, women represented only 28 percent of nursing syndicate members in 1908 and 26 percent in 1911.[11] Most of the hospital employees' organizations were founded and run by men.

The Syndicat du Personnel Non-Gradé was the one notable exception to this pattern: it grew from 27 percent female membership in 1904 to 76 percent in 1908, though the proportion fell to 53 percent by 1911. Despite the SPNG's strong record on female membership, the union's adjunct-secretary Ferdinand Merma complained on several occasions of the women's weak showing at syndicate meetings and of their failure to act in their own best interest. In 1907 the union's Secretary Huyvetter pleaded with the female employees to put an end to their passivity, which implied collaboration with the administration. He urged them instead to join their male colleagues in the struggle for liberty:

> You will thereby be worthy of the title "woman," which means to be a contributor and a teacher, having struggled, suffered, and conquered . . . you will continue the tradition of those sublime women of the people who, in '71, loaded men's guns and were themselves killed with men . . . If

you are "feminine," you will prove that those who claim that you are inferior beings are correct . . . Nurses to arms! Nurses to victory![12]

In the years before the war the women employees continued to disappoint
Huyvetter, ignoring his clarion call for a phalanx of revolutionary female
nurses who would claim their true womanhood by joining their male com-
rades on the barricades of class warfare. Merma and Huyvetter's comments
indicate that the mere presence of large numbers of women in an organization did not ensure that their voices would be heard.

Given the larger context of the history of labor movements in France, it
is hardly remarkable that men dominated the hospital workers' syndicates
and associations. According to historian Madeleine Guilbert, women represented just over five percent of the organized work force in France in
1900, and reached a prewar peak of just under ten percent in 1911, at a
time when their participation in the nonagricultural work force stood at
close to 37 percent.[13] But male dominance of the various hospital employees' organizations was more than just a reflection of the national profile of
organized labor. In the public hospitals of Paris, as well as in Nice, Marseilles, Lyons, and a handful of other large cities where hospital employees'
groups formed, gender issues were at the very center of the unionizing impulse. Controlled by men, these organizations were concerned, in a very
real sense, with the gendered nature of the work they performed.[14] The
nurses' unions attempted to establish a new internal order in the nation's
public hospitals that would preserve the institutions for working-class men
and women alike and establish nursing as a gender-neutral occupation.
In direct opposition to the administrative, governmental, and medical
discourses on the need to feminize and professionalize nursing, these
groups—whether militant or accommodationist—insisted that nursing
was a skilled trade and hence could be practiced by anyone with motivation, training, and aptitude.

The two and a half decades before the First World War saw the establishment of a half dozen or so societies, associations, and syndicates among
the "secondary personnel" of the Paris Assistance Publique.[15] Until 1904,
when the lower-ranking employees broke away from the Association
Amicale du Personnel Hospitalier, organizational efforts centered on ad-
dressing the common grievances of all personnel.[16] The first hospital workers' group to form after the 1884 law authorizing professional trade unions
was the short-lived Syndicat et Union Fraternelle des Sous-Employés et

Infirmiers de l'Assistance Publique, which met for the first (and apparently last) time in the fall of 1891. Established under the banner of Jean Allemane's Parti Ouvrier Socialiste Revolutionnaire, the union stated as its general goal the collective defense of the workers' rights against the "innumerable abuses" perpetrated by the "top-ranking employees of the administration."[17] According to the administrator dispatched to monitor the meeting, the call to action drew only nine employees, all men.

By comparison, the Chambre Syndicale des Infirmiers, Infirmières et Gardes-malades du Departement de la Seine was at least a modest success. Organized in the fall of 1892 and claiming 1,500 members at its peak, the Chambre Syndicale put forth two major goals: to serve as a central employment agency for hospital and private nurses and to "defend the interests of . . . members in the disputes which can arise in the exercise of their functions and to claim their rights in all circumstances."[18] Under the direction of one Louise Coutant—the only woman to take a leadership position in a prewar nurses' syndicate—the organization appears to have functioned primarily as a job exchange, locating suitable positions for its Paris members in municipal hospitals and in private homes. The syndicate required adherents to have a diploma or three years of nursing experience with satisfactory reports, and adamantly refused its endorsement to any nurse whose performance could not be guaranteed.[19]

From the beginning Louise Coutant went out of her way to be conciliatory toward the Assistance Publique administration. "I assure you," she wrote to the AP Director, "that I have never had the desire to enter into struggle with your administration. To the contrary, I hope that later on, seeing how carefully we have prepared our statutes, how rigorously we mean to have them respected, you will one day grant us your trust."[20] But the syndicate's pledge to defend the rights and interests of its members "under all circumstances" made the administration doubt the organization's claims to conciliation. The syndicate, for its part, resorted to sending announcements of meetings to all employees to protect the identity of its members.[21] For a full decade the organization unsuccessfully battled the AP administration for recognition and for access to records and performance evaluations of the nursing personnel. The group's struggle with the administration took its toll, and by 1901, enrollment had dropped to 144.[22] In the spring of 1902, Coutant regretfully informed the AP that the syndicate was abandoning its efforts in the Parisian institutions and, from then on, was devoting its energies solely to placing nurses in provincial hospitals and homes.[23]

Echoing the language of reformers like Bourneville and Hamilton, Coutant blamed the syndicate's failure in part on the employees themselves who, she claimed, lacked the level of dedication and training essential to the survival of lay nursing. Ultimately, however, she held the administration responsible for refusing to support the syndicate's reform efforts. In her last letter to the AP, Coutant wrote bitterly that the "Administration, with puerile fear, did not want to recognize us and that was as regrettable for it as for us."[24] What could have been a collaborative effort aimed at improving the lay nursing staff ended at an impasse that benefited no one. It was the administration, not the syndicate, she argued, that forced the conclusion that the material and professional interests of the nursing personnel were fundamentally at odds with those of the Assistance Publique.

The syndicate met with considerable resistance from hospital administrators, who saw in the organization a potentially powerful threat to their authority. Even Bourneville, whose own suggestions for reform closely resembled those of the new organization, and who minced no words in voicing frustration at the AP administration's recalcitrance, distrusted the political agenda of the nurses' syndicate. Although he approved of the group's potential for promoting professional training among the hospital personnel and finding positions for private nurses, he had strong misgivings about its function as the voice of collective action in the city's public institutions. The hospital and asylum nurses' situation, he argued, "is not at all the same as that of workers, vis-à-vis their employers." Whereas most workers had no intermediary bodies representing their rights and grievances to their bosses, the nurses had recourse to the municipal and departmental councils, both of which always had the nurses' best interests in mind.[25] Bourneville and most administrators were unable or unwilling to regard nurses as independent social actors capable of representing their own interests to their superiors.

Predictably, Bourneville's greatest fears centered on the potential threat the syndicates posed to the nationwide laicization of hospital nursing staffs. Several "newspapers hostile to the lay personnel," he observed, had noted that the formation of a syndicate meant that the lay nursing staff would inevitably go on strike, thereby creating an opportunity for the reintegration of the religious sisters. Bourneville dismissed the assertion as absurd: the *surveillantes* were too devoted to their duties to walk out, and the nuns would never take the lower-level *infirmière* positions. Nonetheless, he feared that even the remotest threat of a strike might serve to dissuade provincial hospital administrations from laicizing their staffs.[26]

Although short-lived, the syndicate's very existence and the nature of its demands suggest that the professional life of the hospital nurse had become newly politicized. The organization's desiderata were clearly informed by the chorus of trade-union demands that had grown steadily louder since the legalization of professional associations in 1884. Heading the nursing syndicate's list was the establishment of the twelve-hour day; close behind was a prohibition against arbitrary termination of employment. In a further bid for control over their working lives, the members of the Chambre Syndicale demanded a guarantee that personnel holding a nursing diploma be given preference in hiring and promotion decisions.[27] The group also stressed material improvements such as the replacement of dormitories with individual rooms (especially for the female staff), better food, prohibition against tipping, and salary increases.

Like Coutant's Chambre Syndicale, the Groupement du Personnel Secondaire de l'Assistance Publique underwent a process of radicalization over the course of its rather brief existence. Founded in 1896, the Groupement was the only other employees' organization that attempted to represent the interests of the AP personnel of all ranks. Its original statement of purpose stressed its role as a mutual aid society for members and their families stricken by illness or death, and declared explicitly that the organization "has no trade unionist aspects and in no case will it offer unemployment compensation."[28] Most of the group's activities, at least for the first few years of its existence, appear to have been limited to sponsoring benefit concerts and raffles, and it apparently avoided political activism of any sort. In its apolitical role of friendly society, the Groupement enjoyed the full backing of the Assistance Publique administration. It received an annual subsidy from the administration and even used AP headquarters on the Avenue Victoria as its seat of operations. The association initially enjoyed enormous popularity among the AP staff. According to the Groupement's own statistics, approximately 80 percent of the nonreligious "secondary personnel" paid dues in 1897.[29]

Despite its conciliatory relationship with the AP, the Groupement, led by the Necker pharmacy *surveillant* Auguste Artreux, had the potential to be more than a friendly society. In addition to supplying moral and material aid in times of hardship, the organization also undertook to "study and support all questions that can facilitate the improvement of our well-being and the growth of our administrative situation and to come to the aid of each member by all means in its power and in all situations where its intervention will be deemed necessary."[30] Here was a statement of intent broad enough to include any militant political program that stopped short of a strike.

That potential was exploited when *surveillant* François L'Héritier, editor of the group's newspaper, *L'Infirmier,* took on the controversial issue of the gendered division of hospital work. By the spring of 1899, L'Héritier had staked out an unequivocal position that all nursing positions in men's wards must be filled by male nurses and that women be confined to the women's wards. "For several years there has been an attempt to prove that men are not capable of becoming good nurses, that only women have the necessary aptitude," he wrote in June 1899. "It even appears that the nursing vocation is innate in women."[31] L'Héritier argued that the feminization of nursing positions along the lines of the English model would ultimately hurt the interests of all working-class nurses, male and female, because in its efforts to raise the profession's prestige, administrators would favor middle-class women over the poorer but more experienced existing personnel. He maintained that the growing tendency toward feminization of the profession and the celibacy of its practitioners, as demonstrated in the well-publicized example of the Lyons *hospitalières,* could only lead either to the installation of "lay congregations" or the free rein of "amorous single women."[32] L'Héritier, like so many of his more powerful contemporaries, could not envision single women as responsible social actors outside of a religious context.

Using language common to many labor unions at the time, L'Héritier insisted that the displacement of men by women in the workplace would destroy the home and "double women's burden under the weight of capitalism."[33] The *sous-surveillant* Gabriel Dubois concurred: "The elimination of men in [nursing] positions would have as its goal to reduce further the intellectual level of male nursing recruits, which would fall to the level of common laborers." In the meantime, "the high-ranking women [*gradées*], belonging to a superior social class, will close off advancement for the true working class."[34] Although L'Héritier's near obsession with this theme was unmatched by subsequent hospital labor leaders, his battle cry of "women in women's wards, men in men's wards" ("Les femmes chez les femmes, les hommes chez les hommes") was quickly adopted in the ensuing decade by almost every hospital nurses' union in the country.

It was on this issue of the future of men in nursing that the hospital employees brought their first large-scale and direct challenge to administra-

tive policy. On December 30, 1899, a delegation of at least 250 male and female nurses marched to the Hôtel-de-Ville to protest a municipal council
budget proposal that would require the replacement of men by women in
all services except surgery and the syphilis wards, a policy backed by AP
administrators and many doctors. The group entered the building at mid-
night, only to have the doors to the Council tribunal slammed shut by
frightened legislators. A few minutes later they were admitted to the chamber and allowed to present their grievances. After a brief audience, the
councilmen sent the nurses back to their institutions with vague promises
of due consideration.[35]

The incident revealed the gulf that had opened between the perceived
interests of the hospital authorities and those of the nurses. According to
the feminist newspaper *La Fronde,* the "invasion" of the municipal council
tribunal was spearheaded not by male employees trying to preserve their
jobs, but by female delegates hoping to maintain professional standards.
Declaring that they wanted to remain "nurses and not porters," the women
repudiated the claim of reformist physicians like Bourneville and Marcel
Badouin—with which most Assistance Publique administrators concurred—that feminizing nursing would enhance the profession's prestige.
Instead, they believed that eliminating men from all but a few services
would mean that women would be forced to perform the sort of menial
tasks that degraded their jobs. Without a clear distinction between nursing
duties and domestic service, women would not benefit from a monopoly
on nursing positions.[36]

Alarmed at the Groupement's new confrontational stance, the AP administration refused to grant the nurses material concessions and began to
withdraw privileges previously accorded the organization. Requests for
permission to hold meetings were repeatedly denied, the posting of notices
pertaining to the Groupement was forbidden, notification by the administration of personnel changes was halted, and promises to disburse a 30,000
FF retirement fund already approved by the AP supervisory council were
retracted. Finally, in 1900, the municipal elections brought in a conservative council which promptly denied the organization access to the city government.[37]

The long run of defeats badly compromised support for the Groupement among the staff. "The vitality of the organization, already damaged
by the relative failure of our actions," wrote L'Héritier, "was threatened to
the point where many thought it dead." The weekly journal *L'Infirmier*

ceased publication in the winter of 1900, the result of "the apathy of some colleagues," the "open hostility" of many doctors, and "the accusations issued against it."[38] Internal squabbling and factionalization accelerated the deterioration of the organization. In December 1900 the Groupement, denied permission yet again to hold a meeting in the administration's building, decided to seek membership in the Bourse du Travail, a move that required prefectural authorization as a syndicate. A few months later, the Groupement du Personnel Secondaire de l'Assistance Publique became professional syndicate number 1574. The reconstituted organization counted approximately 2,000 members, less than half the size of the original Groupement.[39]

The syndicate's leadership (which remained intact) insisted that the transformation from association to trade union did not imply political radicalization. Union President Auguste Artreux urged the director of the AP to "see in this syndical association *less a weapon of combat than an instrument of material, moral, and intellectual progress*" [original emphasis].[40] Artreux assured the administration that the move to the Bourse in no way compromised the staff's fundamental allegiance to the patients they served. Above all, the syndicate stressed repeatedly that the personnel would never resort to a strike to achieve its goals. "We are content to affirm that the hospital personnel, poorly fed, poorly clothed, poorly paid, not getting satisfaction for its just demands, will never abandon the patients who are entrusted to them." Even the membership cards explicitly renounced the right to strike.[41]

But the syndicate's assurances elicited no conciliatory gestures from the AP administration. Instead, hospital directors were instructed to forbid the posting of all notices pertaining to the organization, and the personnel was once more denied permission to attend meetings that extended beyond evening curfew. (The *personnel non-gradé* was required to return to the dormitories by 10 P.M. and the *personnel gradé* by 11 P.M.)[42] Backed into a corner, the syndicate finally took an overtly adversarial stance. On April 20, 1901, eight hundred members met at the Bourse du Travail and for the first time admitted that their efforts to collaborate with the administration had failed. In a strikingly forthright resolution, the assembled crowd declared that "they regret the obvious prejudice of the Administration which tends to impede the progress of trade unionism; and that they continue to place their full trust in the provisional syndicate leadership" in its demand for "the complete emancipation of the exploited Assistance Publique [workers]."[43] The hospital administrators had mutated, rhetorically at least, from "grands-pères" of the great "hospital family" into employers and exploiters of working men and women.[44] Both the Assistance Publique administration and the Minister of the Interior refused to recognize the new syndicate.[45]

The political radicalization of the Groupement du Personnel Secondaire marked the beginning of a new era of increasingly hostile relations not only between administration and staff but within the ranks of Paris hospital employees themselves. By 1905 the *Bulletin professionnel des infirmiers et infirmières* listed seven different hospital workers' syndicates and associations, two of which included nurses: the Société Amicale des Surveillants et Surveillantes des Hôpitaux et Hospices de l'Assistance Publique and the Syndicat du Personnel Hospitalier Non-Gradé. Among the non-nursing employee organizations were the Syndicat des Journaliers Non-Professionnels, the Syndicat des Buandiers et Buandières et Lingères, and the Syndicat des Chauffeurs et Mécaniciens. The "principle of solidarity" among the staff of the Assistance Publique, complained the *Bulletin,* had given way to the spirit of factionalism.[46]

The lack of cohesiveness of the hospital staff arose from a growing awareness among the employees that different groups of "secondary personnel" stood in very different relation to the administration and the municipal council and to the reforms those bodies produced. The lower-ranking *personnel non-gradé,* which broke away from the Syndicat du Personnel Secondaire early in 1904 to form the SPNG, adopted a program aimed at transforming Paris's *infirmiers, infirmières,* and *garçons* and *filles de service* into regular municipal workers. The SPNG sought to eliminate all paternalistic administrative prerogatives by instituting complete worker control over free time and, most importantly, by abolishing all payments in kind, including mandatory room and board in the institutions.[47]

At the same time, the higher-ranking *personnel gradé* established the Société Amicale des Surveillants et Surveillantes, which had a completely different political strategy and professional agenda. Carrying on the moderate tradition of the original Groupement, the SASS eagerly sought the support of the Assistance Publique administration and bestowed the honorary presidency of the organization on AP Director Gustave Mesureur. The SASS quickly gained the political backing of the directors and bursars (*économes*) of the individual hospitals and counted among its members a number of prominent physicians.[48]

If the earlier Groupement of all personnel grew out of a sense of common oppression, the SASS and SPNG split arose from an awareness that, common material grievances notwithstanding, the political and professional interests of higher- and lower-ranking employees no longer coincided. The divergent paths cannot be explained by class background. Secondary personnel of all ranks came almost exclusively from the working class and peasantry, and many who first gained employment among the *non-gradés* were eventually promoted to *gradé* positions. The political strategies of the SPNG and the SASS arose, instead, from the groups' different views of the nascent process of professionalization and, consequently, from their different relationships to the organized labor movement.

Like their lower-ranking colleagues, SASS members did not hesitate to take adversarial stands on such material issues as salary increases, weekly days off, improved pensions and benefits, regular promotions, payment of full salary (without deductions for meals or lodging), and the *externat* (independent living outside hospital grounds). But the SASS also voiced its opinion on the definition of professional duties, expressing concern over the dangers of de-skilling and downgrading of positions. Between February 1905 and December 1906 alone, at least 96 *gradé* (*surveillant* and *surveillante*) positions were reclassified as *garçons* and *filles de service* posts in what SASS President Leclerc termed the "methodical elimination of a large number" of supervisory positions.[49] Employees of all ranks protested that they were forced to perform duties outside of their job descriptions, complaining that in some hospitals simple *infirmières* were in charge of entire services while supervisory personnel performed the duties of *filles de service*.[50] The SASS responded with statements specifying the *surveillantes'* administrative and medical responsibilities, and noting the "desirability" of guaranteeing the *surveillant*'s or *surveillante*'s complete authority within a ward or service. Limited as they were, these efforts represented the first attempt on the part of the AP nurses to define the parameters of their professional duties.[51]

Central to nearly all SASS public statements was an insistence on a core ethic of professional altruism that distinguished SASS members from "mere workers." Leaders repeatedly asserted that for the *surveillants* and *surveillantes*, "the devotion to professional duty floats above material interests."[52] Their primary concern always remained "the relief of misery of all those who are entrusted to our care."[53] The best proof of their commitment to professional duty lay in the forceful prohibition against strikes.

"A strike would be a crime," SASS president Mage declared to a "salvo of applause" from the assembled Société members. "Sickness and suffering never go on strike, . . . and those whose mission it is to relieve these miseries must exhibit as much stubbornness and constancy to accomplish it, as does the plague in attacking the disadvantaged."[54] Such altruism stood in marked contrast, Mage claimed, to the beliefs and practices of the *non-gradé* syndicate, whose leaders sought only material gain and political self-aggrandizement.[55]

The SASS practiced a delicate balancing act, hoping to distinguish the *surveillant(e)s* from "mere workers" while simultaneously identifying themselves as members of the working class. Nowhere was the dual character of the supervisory nurse better expressed than in the words of the *surveillante* Marie-Antoinette Guéniot, one of the few women to write for a syndicate publication. In her 1909 tribute to the hospital nurse, Guéniot defined self-sacrifice—the moral currency of religious nursing—as a virtue only when performed by a member of the working class. "To be rich and generous, that is justice," she wrote, "but to be a proletarian and a philanthropist, that is heroism."[56] According to Guéniot, the wealthy had a moral and social obligation to assist the poor and the sick, while the working class did so out of an extraordinary and altruistic commitment to the welfare of their fellow beings. Thus nurses, though decidedly "proletarians," were not merely employees or workers struggling for acceptable work rules and a living wage, but a morally select group dedicated above all to helping the unfortunate.

In this formulation, nurses exhibited characteristics of both workers and professionals: workers in that their economic and political interests remained tied to that of the working class, but professionals in that their material needs were always subordinated to their humanitarian concern for the plight of their patients. Guéniot described the high-ranking nurses as "heroic proletarians," not to associate them with political militancy but to signal the complexity of employer-employee relations in a workplace that was also an institution of public welfare, and where the unit of production was the human patient.

Guéniot was quick to point out, however, that this type of working-class heroism was characteristic only of the higher-ranking hospital employees. Whereas the lower-ranking *personnel infirmier* or *non-gradé* performed duties ranging from the purely manual chores of transporting patients and cleaning to the skilled tasks associated with direct patient care, the elite *personnel surveillant* or *gradé* supervised medical and general services of all kinds and had authority over the *personnel infirmier* under their command. As subordinates in the nursing hierarchy, the *personnel infirmier* naturally identified with the militant politics of the trade union movement, which offered "moral uplift" as well as an agenda that addressed their most urgent material needs. In Guéniot's estimation, the lower-ranking staff understandably found common cause with other laborers in their efforts to oppose the potentially exploitative policies of their employers.

By contrast, the *personnel surveillant,* though emphatically still of the working class, had no need for trade unions or the "moral uplift" they could provide. After all, Guéniot asserted (not quite accurately), many *surveillantes* had university degrees in addition to the diploma offered by the administration, and some could even "rival the functionaries of other state administrations" in educational accomplishment. She maintained that, in fact, many among the *surveillant* personnel found that their interests overlapped more often with those of the hospital administrators or civil servants than with their lower-ranking co-workers.[57] Thus, although Guéniot agreed that secondary hospital personnel of all ranks had material grievances that were most effectively addressed collectively, she resisted the formation of a syndicate among the upper-level staff members and instead embraced the more conciliatory and solidarist-minded Société Amicale (friendly society) of Surveillant(e)s. For Guéniot, the occupational identity of the supervisory nurses was rooted simultaneously in an unshakable solidarity with the "proletarian class" and an explicit affirmation of their transcendent professional allegiance to the welfare of the institution they served. Unlike their lower-ranking colleagues, the first duty of the *surveillant(e)s* was to their patients, not to self-interest. This distinction set them apart fundamentally from the ordinary ranks of "proletarians" from which they had proudly emerged.

The SASS image of the professional nurse was the product of both animosity toward the SPNG and the *surveillants'* and *surveillantes'* urgent need to defend their jobs against the nursing congregations, whose return to the AP hospital wards remained a potential threat until the war. Unlike the professional models put forth by Hamilton in Bordeaux or Bourneville in Paris, the SASS vision of the professional nurse did not emphasize formal training. Aware that increasing numbers of nuns were attending the municipal schools, the SASS downplayed the importance of the professional diploma and stressed the inherent connection between nursing care and family care from which the religious sisters were, by definition, excluded. As Mage noted in 1905,

> the *congréganistes* . . . want to reconquer their place [in the hospitals] at any cost. Adoring today what they rejected yesterday, they are taking courses in our schools and obtaining diplomas. It is up to us to show that it is not enough to possess a parchment [diploma] to be a good nurse. There are certain qualities of the heart that the nun is utterly lacking, that she will never possess . . . her education and her life style being the absolute negation of the family and all that is connected to it.[58]

Family responsibilities prepared nurses for the care of both physical wounds and moral wounds, Mage's successor Leclerc announced at the organization's Fête de la Laicisation in 1905.[59] Mage and Leclerc both recognized that without an essentialist definition of the nurse that excluded nuns, the lay *surveillants* and *surveillantes* might soon find themselves at a professional disadvantage.

But stressing the centrality of family to the professional identity of the nurse could easily play into the hands of those hoping to feminize the field. After all, if the family was the best nursing school, then surely motherhood was its most valuable preparatory course. The SASS position on feminization was ambivalent: its leaders never endorsed or repudiated the principle of feminization. While avoiding any suggestion that women had an *a priori* claim to particular nursing jobs, they acknowledged that important gender differences existed in the current organization of hospital work, and that the SASS would achieve the status and recognition it deserved only with the active involvement of its female adherents. "We [the *surveillants* and *surveillantes*] are the mainspring of the hospital administration," wrote the newly instated SASS President Leclerc in 1906. "You especially, Mesdames les Surveillantes, are the direct intermediaries between the hospital administration and the medical corps." The female *surveillantes* provided the link between the authorities (both the administration and the medical corps) on the one hand, and the ward staff and patients on the other. It was the *surveillantes* who were responsible for upholding administrative regulations in the wards and for following through on all doctors' orders. Patients and their families alike, Leclerc observed, "know only the *surveillante*."[60]

The SASS emphasis on "the family" as the cornerstone upon which nursing should be built also allowed it to make material demands in the name of "the right to support a family." Like the SPNG, the SASS cited the universal right to maintain a private home as the grounds upon which they claimed payment of their complete salaries without deductions for meals or lodging and without needing permission to live outside the institution (*external*).[61] "The realization of this promise," wrote Guéniot in 1907, "would be for us the promised land; it would be an oasis, after the exhaustion of the day." A full salary and a home of one's own were nothing more than the fulfillment of the republican promise of Liberté, Egalité, and Fraternité.[62]

The SASS successfully presented itself to the AP authorities as an organization seeking the amelioration of nurses' working conditions, but less in terms of workers' rights than in the interest of creating an effective public assistance apparatus. The majority of SASS members rejected repeated efforts in 1905, 1906, and 1909 to convert the association into a syndicate, insisting on maintaining a nonadversarial stance toward their superiors and reminding would-be militants that because hospital employees could not make use of the strike, conversion to a syndicate would be meaningless.[63] Not all SASS members agreed with this strategy. In 1909 a handful of male *surveillants* took it upon themselves to organize the Syndicat des Gradés and launched an aggressive campaign to attract members from the Societé. Accusing the SASS of general ineffectualness, the unionists met with angry resistance from the Societé's leaders, who feared both dissension among their 1,400 members and the birth of a new ally of the perennially adversarial SPNG. According to the SASS, the syndicate received little support from the hospital personnel. Yet what little information there is on the syndicate suggests that it became quite active during the war, when it began to present the cases of aggrieved members to the administration, much in the style of the SPNG.[64] The SASS's rejection of the syndicate came at the cost of diverting a considerable amount of its energy to internal political issues and of dividing the allegiances of the hospitals' supervisory staff.

Like the SASS, the Syndicat du Personnel Non-Gradé focused its energies on the improvement of working conditions under the broad banner of "greater individual liberty." The union's original objectives were in fact barely distinguishable in content and in tone from the far more conservative SASS and the earlier Groupement. At the most concrete level, the SPNG demanded the abolition of the requirement that *infirmiers* and *infirmières* sleep in dormitories or on the wards, complete discretion in the use of off-duty hours, ownership of uniforms, and an end to the policy of punishing employees by confinement to their quarters. Demanding "to be considered a professional corporation and not domestic servants," the unionists stressed "the full payment of salaries without deductions and assimilation to workers of the city of Paris." But even these basic material concerns were couched in the altruistic rhetoric of the SASS: "We would like those who come to the hospitals for care to find a personnel with a better situation." In making their material claims, they argued, their concern was less for their own well-being than for that of the patients.[65]

In many respects, the history of the SPNG fits neatly into the history of French trade unionism during the heady days of labor activism of the early twentieth century. Unlike the SASS, the SPNG spokesmen explicitly tied the fortunes of the nursing personnel to the achievements of organized labor. The syndicate's journal, *L'Action,* displayed the slogan "The emancipation of workers can only be the accomplishment of the workers themselves," and its editors portrayed the paper as a link between SPNG members and the larger trade union movement. "A battalion in the proletarian army," the mission statement declared, "we take care of our brothers in arms."[66] The union participated enthusiastically in annual May 1 demonstrations and endorsed strikes by other syndicates throughout the country. Not infrequently, SPNG meetings or public demonstrations closed with a rendition of the "Internationale."

Like the SASS, the SPNG abjured the strike for itself but, characteristically, cast the policy in political rather than moral terms. Ferdinand Merma, adjunct-secretary and later treasurer of the syndicate, explained on more than one occasion that for the nurses "the duty of solidarity" demanded that they remain "in the wards where one cares for those wounded in the fight." The vast majority of patients, after all, came from among the poor or working class, their comrades-in-arms. On at least four occasions, in 1907, 1908, 1909, and 1913, the SPNG went so far as to threaten a strike, but in all four cases the tactic was eventually abandoned.[67] In December of 1912, the SPNG adopted a resolution declaring that although duty prohibited the syndicate from joining the 24-hour general strike, it remained "in solidarity with the organized working class and approves its decisions" and "declares that in the case of war it will conform to the resolutions adopted by the . . . CGT."[68]

Although the SPNG presented itself as a workers' organization committed to ameliorating the condition of all lower-level hospital employees, its leadership was consistently dominated by general service workers. Eugène Duval, secretary of the syndicate, served as a second-class *garçon de service* at the Lariboisière Hospital. (He left his hospital post in December 1904 "at his own request," apparently to become a full-time organizer.) Abadie, who also served as secretary, held the rank of *infirmier* but worked in a general service capacity. Merma, one of the most vocal and powerful of the group's leaders, was a third-class *garçon de service* at the Beaujon Hospital and an *infirmier* (with indeterminate duties) in the CGT clinic.[69]

Recognizing that the syndicate's bargaining position with the administration would be strengthened by a demonstration of the union's support among the nurses who provided direct patient care, the syndicate leadership stressed that the group also included many *infirmiers* and *infirmières soignant(e)s*. In 1911, for example, Merma wrote to the editor of *Le Temps* protesting a doctor's characterization of the SPNG as including "only employees responsible for heavy labor."[70] Merma feared that if the Assistance Publique authorities regarded the SPNG as representing only unskilled laborers, its demand "to be considered a professional corporation" would be ignored. He realized that the doctors and administrators made a clear distinction between care-giving nurses and general service workers, regardless of the SPNG's own organizing strategy.

The SPNG's goal as a professional union of hospital workers and nurses was to carve out a collective identity distinct from the category of the domestic servant. "In all the cities it is approximately the same situation," Duval complained in 1910; "nurses [*infirmiers*] are not recognized as professionals, we are considered less than domestics." Like the SASS, the SPNG's main grievance centered on the personnel's lack of autonomy, and in particular, the administration's lodging and dining policies that denied members their right to a private family. (As of the fall of 1906, almost three-quarters of the *personnel non-gradé* lived in the hospitals or hospices where they worked.)[71] Without a "family life," wrote SPNG Secretary Huyvetter in 1907, "we have no reason to envisage the future."[72] Only domestic servants and religious orders were still expected to sacrifice completely their individual freedom for the convenience of their superiors.

The SPNG took particular exception to administrative policies that curtailed the independence of female staff, policies that clearly invoked the religious life. Secretary Huyvetter argued that by denying young women the right to lodge outside the hospital (externalization), the administration in essence sacrificed the *infirmières'* physical and mental health to ensure "good publicity" for the administration.[73] In other words, he implied, the similarity between female residency requirements and congregational life served the administration's purpose of ensuring the morality of their workers and the legitimacy of their self-sacrificing labor. But female hospital employees were not nuns, and administrative efforts to pretend that they were stood in direct contradiction to women's rights as workers and as human beings. The syndicate never seriously disputed the inherently feminine character of many (though not all) nursing positions. Instead, it sought to bring the *infirmières* out of the category of domestic servants into that of politicized workers. As long as the administration insisted on controlling the private lives of its female employees (who constituted about 64 percent of the *non-gradé* staff in 1906), the status of all secondary personnel remained compromised.

Relations between the SPNG and the administration deteriorated markedly from 1907 on, as the syndicate adopted increasingly militant tactics. On May 1 the union organized demonstrations in favor of "individual liberty," including a call for all personnel to ignore administration rules regulating workers' lives during their off-duty hours. An anonymous report drafted by the AP administration in 1908 noted that the SPNG "is heading more and more toward revolutionary action." By the fall of 1908, the administration reported that Merma had hanged an effigy of AP director Gustave Mesureur in the syndicate headquarters at the Bourse du Travail and had made detailed plans to strike. Whether or not Merma actually had such intentions, no strike was ever called.[74]

Perhaps in response to the syndicate's growing hostility, the Assistance Publique partially conceded the issue of "personal liberty" to the SPNG, but maintained distinctions between male and female workers. In the fall of 1909, AP Director Mesureur proposed a revision of the 1903 regulation that called for, among other things, the *externat* for two-thirds of the hospital's male personnel and one-third of female employees. Acknowledging that the complaints of the hospital personnel simply expressed "the aspirations toward liberty that characterize the current demands of all workers," Mesureur wrote sympathetically that a "malaise" had swept through the ranks of personnel. The employees "do not feel 'at home' in the hospital, and it is of the 'home' that they dream, with its intimacy and relative comfort."[75]

Mesureur grounded his gender-specific policy in cultural notions of men and women's different "natures." Man, he argued, naturally had a "more independent character [and] . . . is more repelled by communal life." Married or single men require their freedom. Women, on the other hand, benefit from the "communal life." In fact, Mesureur could find no reason why an unmarried, childless woman would even want to live outside the hospital. The institution provided companionship and "some of the pleasures of family life." More importantly, the hospital offered young, single women a guarantee of moral protection from the "promiscuities" and other "dangers" that attended life in "some furnished room" in the city.[76]

Mesureur clearly harbored a certain nostalgia for days gone by, when the hospital nurses and other staff still purportedly appreciated the beneficence of their paternalistic employer. "It is not impossible," Mesureur wrote wistfully, "that in the more or less distant future, the opposite tendency will manifest itself among the employees, who will return on their own to the old concept of the hospital-family." The current distaste for communal life stemmed directly and inevitably, the director believed, from the triumph of laicization. For all his support for that project, Mesureur had to admit that in the process something important had been lost; independence and individualism had triumphed over community and solidarity. Distressingly, this trend revealed itself among women as well as among men. Only reluctantly and under great pressure did the AP director accede—and then only partially—to the syndicate's assertion that the hospital nurses and the rest of the secondary personnel, male and female, were no less and no more than workers.[77]

The SPNG's angry response to the proposed AP reforms centered not only on the unequal allotment of the *externat*, but on the introduction of different pay scales for men and women. The new measure stipulated salaries ranging from 600 to 750 francs annually for *filles de services* in four different classes, whereas for men, salaries started at 800 francs for a third-class *garçon de service* and increased to 950 for the highest-ranking *classe exceptionnelle*. The same 200 franc differential was applied to the *non-gradé* nursing personnel (650–800 francs for women, 850–1,000 francs for men).[78] The AP administration, led by the Socialist Heppenheimer (who also sat on the municipal council), defended the disparity on the grounds that the old pay scale "was calculated principally for women" and, as a result, was unfair to male employees whose monetary needs were naturally greater. Whereas women's salaries in AP institutions were comparable or superior to those earned by women in private industry, men could do significantly better outside the hospitals. As a result, the male staff was both unstable and of poor quality.[79]

To the male *non-gradé* personnel, in particular the *infirmiers* who worked in the wards, the introduction of a substantial gender-based salary differential was cause for alarm rather than rejoicing. Still fighting the losing battle to assign all nursing positions in men's wards to men, the SPNG viewed the salary reforms as strengthening the trend toward complete feminization. By 1910 men were losing ground even in the mental hospitals, where physical strength was considered desirable for the nursing staff.[80] Since men and women worked the same number of hours and ran the same risks on the job, one SPNG member reasoned, why should they not receive the same pay? The syndicate, dependent on the support of women who dominated the hospital staff at all but the lowest levels, stressed that men and women together had a fundamental interest in maintaining equal salaries; their fortunes as workers were intrinsically bound to one another.

But not all among the *personnel non-gradé* agreed with this egalitarian strategy for preserving men's jobs. In the fall of 1909, a group of about 600 *garçons de service* withdrew from the SPNG and formed an Association Corporative. Chief among the new "yellow" (administration-backed) association's differences with the SPNG was its rejection of collaboration with female employees and its advocacy of separate lists of demands for men and women, including different salary scales. The Association stressed the need for a "family wage," arguing that all women's work outside the home inevitably led to the destruction of the family and the disintegration of society. The group went beyond the demand to preserve men's nursing positions in men's wards and insisted that "nothing proves that, professionally, we would not be capable of replacing the female nurse in almost all the services."[81]

The male leadership of the SPNG remained steadfast in its opposition to sex-based salary differentials, despite the efforts of the Association Corporative and a similar, short-lived group based at the Hôpital Saint-Louis.[82] Aware that women had potentially more clout with the administration than the increasingly dispensable men, they encouraged their female colleagues to speak out on the issue, and indeed some of the most articulate voices of protest were those of women.[83] Eugénie Reitz, an *infirmière* at the Bicêtre Hospice, argued that women's hospital work was often more difficult and more dangerous than that assigned to men. Women were frequently expected to perform heavy cleaning duties as well as tend to patients, both of which carried the risk of exposure to disease. Men, by contrast, were usually confined to "the rough work" of lifting and transporting supplies and patients and washing laundry. Moreover, she maintained, the assertion that men had greater financial needs was simply false. Every stage of a working woman's life carried dire risks. "Let us assume the woman is married; but what if she is widowed? In that case she will not be spared the urgent demands of life and because she is a woman she may also have to contribute to the support of young children. . . . An unmarried woman may have to provide for old parents left behind in the countryside."[84] The *surveillante* Marguérite Victor, although not personally affected by a measure that applied only to lower-level employees, added simply that "throughout eternity the female hospital personnel has earned the same salaries as the male personnel of the same level; we demand that [this practice] continue because it is just."[85]

With the promulgation of the reforms, the increasingly tense relations between the SPNG and the administration reached the breaking point. In May 1910, about 120 syndicate members, frustrated that the promised salary increases had not been instituted, marched from the Hôtel-de-Ville to the Rue de Bernardins singing the "Internationale" and shouting "Our one hundred sous! . . . Boo [Prefect] de Selves! Mesureur to Charenton [the national mental asylum]!"[86] The syndicate's publication, *L'Action,* launched a scathing campaign against the administration and against the *surveillantes* and *surveillants,* protesting everything from low salaries and spoiled food to the denial of permission to attend a doctor's funeral.[87] Finally, in August 1911, the AP administrators took decisive action against the union and cut off all communication with Duval and Merma. Relations between the syndicate and the administration did not resume until March 1914.[88]

The SPNG leaders presented themselves as the defenders of professional, behavioral, and moral standards among hospital workers in a struggle to repudiate their image as domestic servants in state-run "homes." They called repeatedly for strict enforcement of recruitment standards, asserting that the administration's laxness led directly to the degradation of their profession.[89] According to *L'Action,* applicants for hospital jobs could simply walk in off the street, produce a copy of their police record, and begin work. "The elite personnel, that is to say the majority, suffers from this hasty recruitment that can entail the most unfortunate consequences for the patients." The administration's persistence in hiring these "black sheep" effectively denigrated the entire personnel in the eyes of the public and the patients. The SPNG called for "the meticulous selection of the personnel" and a stringent policy of verifying "the qualifications of candidates."[90]

At the same time as the *personnel non-gradé* worked to raise recruitment standards, they also rejected efforts to transform nursing into an elite profession. They denied that nursing was, or should be, an explicitly feminine occupation requiring a solid educational background, several years of full-time training, and a lifestyle that prohibited marriage or children. The establishment of the Ecole des Infirmières de l'Assistance Publique at the Salpêtrière Hospital (in 1907) appeared to the SPNG as the specter of impending professionalization. Members of the union consistently referred to the Salpêtrière graduates as *Bleues,* alluding in the first instance to their blue uniforms, but undoubtedly also playing on the pejorative term for self-important female intellectuals, *bas-bleus.* While the SPNG applauded the seriousness with which the administration approached the new school and appreciated the prestige accorded its graduates, the educational and social gap between the Salpêtrière students and the majority of the existing nursing staff, as well as the school's status as a single-sex institution, made conflict inevitable. Even those nurses who had already received a diploma from one of Bourneville's older programs could not compete with the two-year, full-time training experience of the Salpêtrière graduates.[91]

The SPNG's vision of the future of hospital nursing—a future in which all nurses joined their fellow laborers in a struggle against their employers for greater independence and a fair salary—differed fundamentally from the model of nursing espoused by the Salpêtrière school. Despite the protestations of one Salpêtrière student that they were "all members of the same professional corps—freely chosen" and that they all "filled the same noble mission chosen and loved above all for its own grandeur despite its difficult constraints," it is doubtful that the readers of the syndicalist paper where the statement appeared accepted the sincerity of the assertion of solidarity. One member of the SPNG complained bitterly that although the *Bleues* preached common cause with their "sisters in misery," their presence in the hospitals only divided the nursing ranks. "Those who pretend to have the same feeling as I, should propagate them inside rather than outside the syndical organization, which will never be solid as long as individuals are divided."[92] At best, the *Bleues* would spend a few years among the *non-gradé* personnel and then move into the ranks of *surveillantes* or into private duty nursing. At worst, their presence in the hospitals signified the complete professionalization and feminization of the field. As the Lyons syndicate president observed in 1912, schools like the Salpêtrière demanded "certain educational abilities to enter, abilities that we do not have and that many of us do not and will not have the possibility of acquiring." If the future of nursing lay with the *Bleues,* it was a future that excluded the SPNG and the majority of the existing working-class personnel.[93]

The efforts of nurses and other hospital secondary personnel to organize on behalf of their rights as skilled workers were most visible in the capital city, where the sheer size of the Assistance Publique staff and its early laicization made it the logical center of collective activity. But the leaders of the Parisian syndicates, especially the SPNG, recognized that the future of lay nursing depended on their ability to address the problems that confronted hospital employees throughout the country. In June 1907, the hospital workers' syndicates of seven French cities organized a national Federation of Hospital Workers (Fédération des Travailleurs Hospitaliers), under the auspices of the CGT. Over the course of the next decade and a half, the federation articulated a clear agenda centering on the need to protect nurses from the dual threats presented by the religious nursing sisters and the elite, well-educated, unmarried *Bleues.*

In theory, the federation sought to bring together representatives of all positions from all types of hospitals. In 1908, the organization changed its name to Fédération des Services de Santé (FSS), so as not to exclude "laboratory assistants, doctors, private nurses, etc." who might not feel welcome in a group that appeared to be organized by "craft" rather than by "industry."[94] But for an organization affiliated with the CGT, diversity was hard to come by and the federation remained dominated by the more radical, lower-ranking personnel. Although the small Syndicat du Personnel Gradé of Paris joined the FSS in 1909 and, after much heated debate, the Syndicat de Médecine Sociale (an organization of Socialist doctors) was admitted, almost all of the nineteen syndicates that had affiliated by the beginning of the war hailed from hospitals and asylums in large towns and drew their members from among the *non-gradé personnel.*[95]

A month after its establishment, the federation, under the leadership of the SPNG's Eugène Duval, met in Paris for its first annual convention. Over the course of the five-day meeting, syndicate delegates from the capital and six provincial cities—Carcassonne, Toulouse, Toulon, Lyons, Nice, and Montpellier—compiled a list of grievances and demands that they hoped would form the basis of a nationwide campaign to improve the lot of all salaried hospital and asylum workers and to shape the future of the nursing profession. The federation members agreed to reject all administrative offers of civil-servant status on the grounds that "none of its members enjoys the so-called advantages accorded civil servants."[96] Instead, the syndicates strove for legal recognition under the 1884 law on professional syndicates, and the guarantee of such basic labor rights as representative councils of discipline, a weekly day off, and the application of the Millerand-Colliard Law on the ten-hour work day.[97]

Above all, the FSS aimed to improve the quality of the country's nursing personnel while preserving the profession's ties to the organized labor movement. The solution to the problem of poor recruitment and incompetence lay in bypassing administrative and government authorities alike by creating professional training programs at *bourses du travail* (labor union halls) throughout the country. The *bourse* courses would serve the dual purpose of seizing control of the training process from those administrative authorities who opposed laicization or who favored elite, English-style nursing schools, and drawing lay personnel into the *bourses*, where they might be encouraged to join a syndicate. Focusing on practical techniques of hygiene, antisepsis, and treatment, the classes would be organized expressly to accommodate the exhausting schedule of a full-time worker with a family. In cities like Lyons, where the existing, full-time, all-women's nursing school admitted only religious sisters and private-duty nurses, courses at the *bourse du travail* represented the lower-level staff's only hope for professional improvement or accreditation.[98]

The success of the *bourse* instructional program depended on two essential factors: the support of doctors and surgeons who would volunteer to teach the courses, and the creation of a diploma valid in hospitals throughout the country. The former presented little problem for the federation. Despite widespread resistance to laicization among hospital physicians, all delegates could point to at least a handful of practitioners willing to instruct lay personnel for an hour or so a week. Moreover, the syndicates had a history of trying to form alliances with the hospital medical staff against the administration.[99]

The establishment of a national diploma, however, presented a formidable challenge. It required cooperation among innumerable hospital administrations under the direction of the national government, a step toward centralization that was unlikely to occur in the foreseeable future. Moreover, the syndicate delegates themselves were wary of excessive government intervention in the training process. Emile Peillod, a laundry worker who organized and served as general secretary of the Syndicat des Infirmiers et Similaires des Hospices Civils de Lyon, warned that if the state were granted a prominent role in organizing the profession, the result would likely be a network of nursing schools similar to those already set up in Lyons and in the Salpêtrière Hospital in Paris. In that case, most union members would be unable to get diplomas. Few staff members could afford to take two full years off from their paid employment to attend the programs. Instead, the FSS delegates wanted a limited "national program" of practical courses that would be organized by the personnel with the support of a few doctors. The certificate issued by these programs was to be recognized as proof of competence in institutions throughout the country.[100] Even with the backing of some physicians, however, the syndicates never were able to exert sufficient political pressure at either the local or national level to establish a uniform set of training standards and a national certificate for hospital personnel. When the Ministry of Hygiene issued a decree in 1922 creating a national diploma for nurses, Peillod's fears were realized: no *bourse du travail* student could qualify.[101]

According to the FSS, the biggest obstacle to the improvement of the nurses' and hospital workers' material and professional situation remained the powerful presence of the nursing sisterhoods in all but a few provincial towns. The FSS delegates to the organization's annual conference freely admitted that the process of laicization had been at best only a partial success. "The initial fault can be traced to the different hospital and asylum administrations which appear to take pleasure in the poor recruitment of their personnel," explained Peillod.[102] Without sufficient training programs and rigorous recruitment standards, the lay nurses would inevitably prove to be inferior to the experienced religious nurses they were assigned to replace. Similarly, Ferdinand Merma noted with evident disgust that in Cambrai, where untrained lay personnel had been hastily brought in to replace the existing nursing order, even a Socialist municipal councilman had declared that only nuns were capable of caring for the sick.[103] As long as the nuns remained in positions of authority, the syndicate members' capacity to force administrative reforms remained severely curtailed. "That which particularly makes it a necessity for us to pursue the laicization of the hospitals," wrote FSS Secretary Duval in 1911, "is the state of inferiority in which the lay employees in the non-laicized hospitals are held. We must work arduously for laicization, since as long as there is a religious personnel next to us, we will only be a secondary personnel."[104] The FSS passed annual resolutions and orchestrated several meetings with the officials in the Ministry of Labor urging laicization.

Ultimately, however, the Fédération's campaign to replace all *congréganistes* with lay nurses failed. Emile Peillod blamed the defeat on the provincial syndicates, which had not organized effectively around the issue.[105] He also condemned the persistent opposition of the powerful doctors' syndicates, whose members continued to back the religious sisterhoods. The antiparliamentarian Merma held the national government responsible by its refusal to coordinate serious professional training programs for all lay nurses.[106] Wherever the blame lay, the fact remained that outside of Paris and a few other cities, the laicization of nursing staffs had little popular appeal or political momentum.

In the decade before the First World War, lay hospital employees of various ranks and political inclinations struggled to establish themselves as bona fide skilled workers and as public servants with specific moral obligations. But the political and cultural forces militating against the inclusion of hospital nursing among the skilled trades were simply too great. Leaders of the various groups that organized during this period found themselves caught in the impossible bind of supporting the improvement of recruitment standards while opposing the feminization of the occupation, at a time when the latter principle was widely held to be the cornerstone of elevating the status of the field. They insisted on nurses' right to an independent home and to the material wherewithal to make such a home life viable, while the dominant voices of both tradition and reform called for a celebration of the communal—if not congregational—spirit of hospital nursing work. The members of the FSS and its constituent organizations were forced to battle simultaneously against the weakness of the syndicalist movement in general, the continued dominance of religious nursing outside Paris, the national government's increasingly outspoken preference for a feminized hospital nursing staff, and reformers' predilection for an elite, feminized model of professional nursing. Without the numbers or the political clout to take on all these issues simultaneously, the syndicalists remained powerless to affect the fundamental conditions that shaped their working lives.

5

The Nursing Profession
in World War I

"Women are drawn, by their nature, toward aiding the military
wounded. . . . In truth, what a small distance women must travel
to become nurses."

—CÉSAR LEGRAND, *L'ASSISTANCE FÉMININE EN TEMPS
DE GUERRE* (1907)

It is a common assumption among modern scholars and contemporary
observers alike that the First World War marked a major turning point in
the history of nursing. With the beginning of hostilities in the summer of
1914, tens of thousands of women from all social classes rushed to volunteer
in the hospitals and ambulances of the belligerent nations. French
women were no exception. Installed in military and auxiliary medical facilities
throughout the country, this new army of nurses quickly won widespread
public acclaim. Reports of their bravery and devotion under the
most adverse conditions were featured in newspapers and public speeches;
their ordeals became the stuff of ballads and romantic fiction. Cast as a
twentieth-century cross between the Virgin Mary and Joan of Arc, the image
of the young wartime nurse appeared on placards, postcards, and in
the pages of popular magazines.

Suddenly the nursing profession was catapulted into the realm of the
most venerable functions that a refined, educated woman could hope to
perform. No longer was it regarded, in the words of one "doctoresse" writing
in 1916, as a job that fell "between that of a children's nursemaid and a
domestic servant. . . . From one day to the next . . . the care given to the
wounded and sick appeared to women from all social ranks as the most
noble service that they could offer their country."[1] Or, as a writer for the
Revue des deux mondes observed, "the war accomplished what a century of
effort could not; it promoted the role of the nurse to one of dignity."[2]

One problem with this type of contemporary assessment is that it is based heavily on propagandistic sources. For example, the repeated claims of the societies of the Red Cross that serving as a nurse had become the French woman's highest aspiration, or the Bishop of Orléans' insistence that nurses were "the actual presence of la Patrie" to the wounded soldiers, say more about the gendered character of patriotic fervor than about the changing status of the nursing profession.[3] But the heroic, self-sacrificing, eternally maternal nurse was not the only stereotype of the Red Cross volunteer to emerge during the war. As historian Margaret Darrow has shown, formulaic contemporary accounts produced two distinct images of the wartime nurse: in contrast to the "true" nurse, "the angel of mercy and devoted surrogate mother to the *petit poilu*," stood the "false" nurse, more interested in romance and self-aggrandizement than in sacrifice and self-abnegation. "Instead of supporting the masculine war," Darrow writes, "the false nurse tried to hijack it, to undermine the virile national regeneration that was the justification of the war and its ultimate purpose." The false nurse sought glory for herself, the true nurse sought glory for France through service to French soldiers.[4]

The second weakness of both contemporary and modern accounts of wartime nursing is that they presuppose an undifferentiated professional category of "nurse" that simply did not exist in France. The nursing corps that staffed the thousands of military, temporary, and auxiliary hospitals of the war era was comprised of women and men from a wide range of social and professional backgrounds: trained nurses recruited by the army's Service de Santé, career military nurses (male and female), enlisted men assigned to nursing units, well-trained and minimally trained Red Cross volunteer nurses, and members of religious congregations. Too often, the history of nursing in France during the First World War is conflated with the history of the Red Cross volunteer.[5] While the Red Cross nurses are clearly a vital part of the history of nursing, their experiences—and the veneration (and disparagement) heaped upon them—bore little relation to the fortunes of trained career nurses. The difference became starkly apparent in the aftermath of the war. When the armistice was signed in November 1918, most of the volunteer nurses quickly abandoned the nursing profession. They had no intention of embarking on a new career; they had simply wanted to contribute to the war effort.

Far from legitimizing a once marginalized and undervalued profession, the public acclaim for the wartime nurses served to blur the definition of the professional nurse, equating the patriotic young volunteer who had completed three months of instructional classes with the veteran professional with years of training and experience. For example, Madame Béthonod, a wartime volunteer in a Lyons hospital, began her service performing "humble and laborious" duties washing dishes and sheets. Soon, however, she was tending to patients in the wards, and shortly thereafter she was "put in charge of running the entire hospital."[6] As public-health nurse Anne Malterre-Barthe has recently noted, "the lesson of the War served to demonstrate that a quasi-benevolent personnel, very quickly trained, 'recommended' or offering proof of qualities of sacrifice, was worth as much as trained nurses."[7] During the World War I period, nursing ability was reduced once again to a natural attribute of womanhood. In venerating nurses, the public paid tribute not to women's skill or expertise, but to their patriotism expressed through their inherently feminine talent for nurturing.[8]

While journalists, politicians, writers, and many wartime nurses themselves actively promoted stereotypical images of the "true" and "false" nurse based on notions of "true" and "false" feminine patriotic service, career nurses and nursing reformers promulgated their own definitions of "true" and "false" nurses. They struggled to establish clear boundaries between "genuine" nurses with years of formal training and practical experience and women who served temporarily—perhaps even opportunistically—as nurses. Both Paul-Louis Lande and Anna Hamilton, for example, repeatedly voiced their scorn for the Red Cross "ladies" who, after three months of classes, received a diploma that permitted them to serve as nurses in auxiliary military hospitals. Lande, Hamilton, and others recognized that the prominence of Red Cross nurses in the wartime hospitals would ultimately diminish, rather than raise, the profession's status.

The First World War did mark a turning point in the history of nursing in France, but perhaps not the same turning point that the tendentious, patriotic, often propagandistic literature of the period would have us believe. If the spectacle of upwards of 100,000 women from all social classes flocking to serve as nurses for la Patrie demonstrated that women's special aptitudes could be attached fruitfully to the state, it also showed that this attachment was based not on nursing as a skilled medical profession, but rather as charity work or patriotic motherhood.[9]

The presence of female lay nurses in military hospitals was an innovation of the early twentieth century. Until 1908, all hospitals under the control of the Service de Santé Militaire of the Ministry of War were staffed by male *infirmiers* or by members of various nursing congregations, particularly the Sisters of Charity of Saint Vincent de Paul. In 1903 religious sisters ran the wards of eleven out of the nation's thirty-three military hospitals. The laicization of these institutions (in 1903 for most naval establishments and 1904–05 for facilities belonging to the army) entailed the replacement of hundreds of congregational women by male members of the regular military.[10]

Though ultimately successful, the turn-of-the-century campaign to oust the nursing sisters from the military hospitals met with considerable resistance from the national government. State officials expressed reservations reminiscent of the laicization struggles in Paris, Lyons, and Bordeaux. "I believe there is reason to maintain the status quo," Minister of War General Zurlinden responded to a proposal for laicization by the Congrès des Libres-Penseurs Français et de la Fédération de la Libre-Pensée. The presence of the nursing sisters "is a sure moral safeguard, *and no other help could be less costly than theirs*" (original emphasis).[11] As late as 1902, with the anticlerical campaigns of Désiré Bourneville and Prime Minister Emile Combe running at full throttle, the Minister of War backed a parliamentary amendment suppressing the effort to replace the religious sisters with lay nurses, maintaining that "the male and female nurses intended to replace the sisters are not yet trained in sufficient numbers."[12] Despite the resistance of the War Ministry, however, the government-sponsored anticlerical activism of the early twentieth century, which ultimately led to the 1905 law separating Church and state, brought with it the dismissal of all religious nurses from the nation's military hospitals.

Although laicization clearly pleased anticlerical politicians like Bourneville (whose journal, *Le Progrès médical,* gleefully recorded the termination of every contract between the Ministry of War and the nursing congregations), the move left the wards under the sole control of a corps of male *infirmiers* whose reputation was uneven at best. Dr. Granjux, writing in the military medical journal *Le Caducée,* noted that troops and officers alike complained of "the professional ignorance of the military *infirmiers* and the defective or insufficient care that results from it." Even the political press "asked in the name of the families for the cessation of this condemnable state of affairs."[13] According to the *Gazette des hôpitaux,* the men who served in the hospitals ranged in professional background from "farmer," "carter," and "watchmaker" to "notary clerk or a lawyer." The vast majority were "common laborers far more than nurses." The director of the Service de Santé himself lamented that every year the military nursing ranks were filled by men from all walks of life and who possessed absolutely no training.[14] The abysmal quality of the male military nurses eventually led the Ministry of War to support the wartime recruitment of divinity students who were otherwise exempt from the obligatory two-year military service.

Haphazard recruitment made the already difficult task of training the *infirmiers* even more challenging. This situation was further complicated by an 1893 statute mandating that all *infirmiers,* regardless of their actual function, were to be given complete instruction. Thus the *infirmiers de visite* (who provided patient care in the wards) received the same training as the *commis d'écritures* (clerks) and the *infirmiers d'exploitation* (who performed custodial duties and other general labor). Proper instruction for so many men required the full-time services of a doctor for an entire year, a forfeiture of medical expertise that few wartime hospitals could afford.[15]

The laicization of the nation's military hospitals not only revealed the inadequacies of the existing male nursing corps, but it also eliminated any female presence in the wards. After the nursing congregations were dismissed, most state-run military institutions accepted lay women as laundry and kitchen workers, but none allowed women in the wards themselves. The military hospital remained strictly male terrain. It was only the experience of the war that fully legitimized the female presence in the military hospitals, transforming the bedside of the wounded or sick *poilu* into a distinctly feminine space.[16]

The decision to exclude women from the wards generated criticism from the very moment that the first military hospitals were laicized. Dr. Félix Regnault, an editor of the Paris-based *Bulletin professionnel des infirmières et gardes-malades* and co-author with Anna Hamilton of an abridged version of her thesis, lamented in 1905 the "serious gap" that resulted from "the absence of any type of feminine care" in the wards. Others maintained that an exclusively male military nursing corps was proof of France's failure to enter the era of modern health care, a charge levied frequently by advocates of extended, formal training for nurses. Bordeaux medical student Roger Colomb wrote in a widely-publicized 1903–04 study of the "role of the woman in aiding wounded and sick soldiers," that France had fallen shamefully behind England, Germany, Austria, Russia, and even Japan in building a competent corps of female nurses capable of serving in military hospitals, especially during a war.[17]

But arguments favoring the introduction of female lay nurses into military hospitals extended far beyond the pragmatism of ensuring an adequate number of nurses, improving the overall quality of the nursing corps, or of competing with other nations. Using language and images that would become commonplace during the war, advocates maintained that the presence of women—symbolic mothers and sisters—in the hospitals was crucial to the well-being of the troops. Referring to the soldiers as "those grown children, who, if they hadn't been drafted, would have maternal care," the Parisian daily newspaper *Le Matin* insisted in 1907 that the military hospitals had an obligation to somehow replace that care. "How can that be done if not through employing women who alone can evoke the family, the intimacy of the home?" the commentator asked. Women had a "special skill," an "incomparable, natural aptitude for nursing."[18] Only a woman could recreate the home in the hospital, and no venue could duplicate the healing power of the home. A man, however devoted or well-intentioned, wrote the editor of the *Bulletin professionnel des infirmières et des gardes-malades* in 1908, "will never know how to find the words of affectionate pity" or how to demonstrate "that meticulous solicitude at all times that a woman brings to those who suffer." Far from being unwelcome interlopers in exclusively male institutions, women, by virtue of their sex alone, were crucial to both the psychological and the physical processes of healing and thereby essential to the strength of the French military. As one Emile Gilbert asserted at a gathering of Red Cross nurses in 1902: "Instinctively, you possess the quality of the genuine nurse, for, as Michelet has . . . said, 'Woman is true medicine.'"[19] Michelet's (and Gilbert's) words bring added significance to Anna Hamilton's statement in 1900 that (reformed) nursing would "soon constitute the true medicine of women."[20] For Hamilton, women would make their vital contribution to medical advancement in their capacity as trained professionals. For Michelet and Gilbert, the essentialized woman was, by nature, a healing force.

Widespread belief in women's natural capacity to nurse certainly helped them to gain access to the military wards, but as a basis for legitimizing female army nursing it would prove to be, at best, a mixed blessing. The wartime experience would soon reveal that the strong essentialist strain in many arguments favoring the introduction of lay nurses in the army hospitals often subverted pleas for the primacy of thorough training and practical experience. In so doing, it moved nursing further away from the status of "profession" and closer to that of feminine charity work.

The Minister of War's 1907 decision to introduce lay women into military hospitals met with almost universal approval. "All the military doctors will see with satisfaction expert and devoted women coming to assist them," predicted the Bordeaux doctor and nursing reformer Paul-Louis Lande.[21] The eminent Paris doctor Maurice Letulle called the move a "remarkable social revolution," and the military doctor Granjux added that "this reappearance of women in the military hospitals" was the product of "a very high humanitarian sentiment." Members of the military medical establishment added only two conditions to their laudatory appraisal of the 1907 announcement: they insisted that the new nurses be "directly and exclusively subordinate" to the doctors, and that the creation of a new corps of female nurses "not compromise the organization of the male military nursing corps."[22]

The role anticipated for the new lay military nurses was limited from the outset. The women would care for the sick and wounded in the hospital wards, but they would not serve at or near the front, where the "fatigue" and "risk" would certainly prove to be beyond the capacity of female strength. In the event of war, their service would be confined to evacuation hospitals, institutions located in the interior, and other "second-line" facilities. (This last restriction was lifted early in 1917, when most of the male nurses serving in medical units at the front were drafted to serve in combat troops.)[23] The editor of the *Bulletin professionnel des infirmières et des gardes-malades* cautioned aspirants to the new positions that "the role of the military nurse will be more precisely the role once played by the *religieuses,* rather than that of the nurses in the civilian hospitals." Medical students and male nurses would apply all dressings and bandages; even the bulk of the general patient care would be provided by the *infirmiers.*[24] Women would most likely find themselves in supplementary roles, performing tasks related to patient care (such as distributing food) that the male personnel would not do. Not even the staunchest supporters of the feminization of nursing and of the introduction of lay nurses into the military hospitals envisioned any radical changes in the organization or administration of military medicine. The participation of women in institutions associated with war remained peripheral.

Once the decision to admit women had been made, government officials, and specifically the Ministry of War, were faced with the not insignificant problem of identifying and recruiting the new personnel. Anyone who had followed the turbulent history of the laicization of hospitals in Paris and in cities throughout the country would have been only too aware of the difficulties involved in finding adequately trained lay women to replace the experienced religious sisters. The Minister of War admitted in 1905 that although he supported the idea of female lay nurses in principle, such a reform could not take place for several years, given that "in effect, that personnel had not yet been trained in France."[25]

As a series of international crises ratcheted the tension levels in Europe to ever higher levels, political pressure to improve the nation's preparedness for war mounted steadily. Finally, the War Ministry proposed a national competition, set for April 1908, among graduates of "approved" nursing schools (the criteria for this status were never specified) to fill an unspecified number of slots in the French army hospitals.[26] Women who passed the exam would become eligible for service in any of the army's hospitals and would be called up as positions became available.

The nationwide announcement of the competition brought an overwhelming response, despite the fact that the pay scale for the new lay military nurses averaged about fifty to sixty francs less than the salaries allotted to civilian *surveillantes* in Paris municipal hospitals.[27] Between 400 and 500 candidates registered by the March 15 deadline, although nearly three-quarters were eliminated immediately for failure to meet the age, health, and training requirements set out by the Ministry of War. Out of the approximately 120 women who took the exam, about 40 were deemed "admissible," and fewer than ten were accepted for employment in 1908. To nursing reformers like Anna Hamilton, Paul-Louis Lande, and Félix Regnault, who championed the cause of trained, female, lay nurses, the mere fact that the national nursing competition required substantial formal training constituted a triumph. Experience, enthusiasm, and a suitably obedient and gentle demeanor would not suffice to earn the title of military nurse. The state's first direct recruitment of female nurses was based solely on a demonstration of aptitude and training, criteria that boded well for the future of the profession.[28]

In December 1908, the Chamber of Deputies approved the funds necessary to create sixty positions for female military nurses.[29] Out of a total military nursing corps that ran in the thousands, the number of places set aside for trained lay women was modest indeed. It did mark, however, what many hoped was the beginning of a new era, in which professional nursing would be integrated into the military and in which women, as trained and paid experts—rather than as volunteers or as *religieuses*—would become an essential part of the state's wartime effort.

But even before the competition took place, a problem arose that would plague military nursing throughout the war. In the early spring of 1908, the Bordeaux-based *La Garde-malade hospitalière* (France's most widely circulated professional nursing journal) learned that the military planned to allow Red Cross "ladies" to serve three-month-long *stages* in the wards of Val-de-Grâce, the Parisian hospital and training center for military medicine run by the Service de Santé. The move was ostensibly intended to grant practical experience to Red Cross nurses, who otherwise had little access to functioning hospital wards. The Minister of War insisted that the volunteer nurses constituted only temporary staff and that eventually they would be replaced by *infirmières officielles*.[30]

The Red Cross societies apparently chose to interpret the decision differently. Speaking before the annual general assembly of the Société de Secours aux Blessés Militaires (SSBM), the oldest of the three organizations that comprised the French Red Cross, the society's president, the Marquis de Voguë, noted proudly that "our Lady nurses have been called to offer their care to the sick and wounded of the army in the military hospitals, and perform there a military service." Together with the other two Red Cross organizations, the Association des Dames Françaises (ADF) and the Union des Femmes de France (UFF), the SSBM volunteers would serve on the Val-de-Grâce wards without first taking an exam or otherwise proving their merit.[31]

Advocates of nursing professionalization were outraged. The editors of *La Garde-malade hospitalière* expressed their "stupefaction" that whereas only a handful of "trained professionals" who had "proved themselves" in a competitive exam were to be admitted, the military had "opened the doors of its instructional hospital to a personnel recruited *autrement*." The Minister of War's decision constituted "an offense, if not an iniquity, with regard to all the dedicated women" who had dutifully registered for the competition. "In the name of all true nurses" the journal demanded that no such nefarious precedent be established. The move could only compromise future reform of the army hospitals.[32]

The hostile response of *La Garde-malade hospitalière* to the presence of

Red Cross nurses in the military hospitals sounded an opening salvo in what would become the defining battle for professional hospital nursing in France. In many ways, the Red Cross "lady-nurse"—unpaid, haphazardly trained, and yet extolled for her charity, devotion, and good will—represented everything that the advocates of rigorous training and strict professional standards opposed. To reformers like Hamilton and Lande, the Red Cross nurse stood as the very antithesis of a professional; to the volunteer, nursing was an avocation, perhaps even a passion, but it was not a career. Her legitimization by the state, in this case by the Ministry of War, only served to uphold the still widespread belief that "from one day to the next any woman, because she had helped her father, her brother, her husband or her child during an illness, could become a good nurse."[33] In the minds of the reformers, women were not, as the Red Cross societies' ethos seemed to maintain, necessarily born nurses.

Critics of the Red Cross nurses argued that the "society ladies" who constituted the vast majority of the organizations' members during the prewar years treated nursing as a diversion or hobby, rather than a vocation or profession.[34] Catherine Elston, *directrice* of the Tondu Hospital in Bordeaux and temporary *directrice* of the Military and Civil Hospital at Elbeuf, praised the particular Red Cross nurses serving at that institution by contrasting them with their colleagues: "They do not come to the hospital by caprice, when the desire to come seizes them," she observed. Instead, "they rush up when they are needed and then they submit themselves to [performing] all the tasks."[35] The American nursing leader Lavinia Dock commented in 1907 that the "ladies" exhibited "an enthusiastic craze for volunteer nursing."

> Dressed in a nurse's uniform, society women, mothers of families, teachers, and school-girls delight in taking "courses" of which there is (sic) an extraordinary number . . . [V]isiting dispensaries to "do dressings" . . . is the especial fad, and one can read pages of sentimental gush (some of it . . . written by doctors) over the admirable devotion of the women who thus desert their social engagements to attend the consultations and assist in the minor surgery of out-patient departments.[36]

Nursing had become an attribute of genteel femininity, a fashionable, even glamorous way for wealthy women to endow their leisure time with social value.

Much of the criticism of the French Red Cross nursing corps during the prewar years centered on training and attitude. Summarizing the most common complaint, Félix Regnault wrote that "the instruction offered by these various [Red Cross] societies can only produce *secouristes* . . . , persons capable of applying a dressing, warding off fainting, etc., but not nurses caring for fever patients or directing a ward."[37] Lavinia Dock complained that the Red Cross training programs remained "superficial" and that the societies made no effort to establish authentic "schools for professional nurses."[38]

Indeed, most of the Red Cross nursing programs did fall short of the standards set in Bordeaux and Lyons and by the Ministry of the Interior in its national circulars of 1899 and 1902. Instruction, which usually took place at a dispensary or small hospital set up by a particular society, generally consisted of theoretical and practical courses as well as some hands-on experience. Schools attached to dispensaries put students to work treating the usually indigent people who came in for out-patient treatment. Those who had access to a hospital accompanied and occasionally assisted the doctors on their rounds.

The chief weakness of the Red Cross nursing schools in the eyes of those promoting formal nursing training was that the complete program leading to a first-degree diploma lasted, on average, only three to six months. (As with public nursing schools, there were no set standards and no minimum national requirements for granting a nursing diploma.) The Dispensaire-Ecole des Dames Infirmières, a school run by the SSBM in Lyons, consisted of lectures and part-day sessions attending patients in the dispensary. After three months, students who passed a written, oral, and practical exam, which tested only the woman's ability to bandage a mannequin and change the dressing on a patient, were issued a nursing diploma. Léonie Chaptal, the prominent social Catholic public health reformer, recalled that in order to receive her Red Cross certificate around the turn of the century, she had only to serve three months in a dispensary and pass an exam consisting chiefly of detailed questions about the skeletal system. Even the *American Journal of Nursing* noted that "it seems that the French societies of women of the Red Cross, who possess influential social position and money, cherish fixed ambitions to act as nurses in military hospitals, but without any intention of submitting themselves to the nurse's arduous training."[39]

Physicians and nursing reformers, for their part, charged that the aspiring nurses showed excessive and inappropriate enthusiasm for acquiring sophisticated knowledge of anatomy, physiology, and medicine in general. In other words, the Red Cross nurses did not observe the professional boundary between doctors and nurses. "The Red Cross ladies are becoming quite rivals for doctors now," Anna Hamilton observed in 1910, "and . . . the Paris doctors are beginning to resent their ways."[40] Paris municipal nursing school professor Dr. Paul Cornet complained that the Red Cross volunteers suffered from "exaggerated . . . professional aspirations." Rather than contenting themselves with observing and helping with patient care in the wards, these women too often insisted on attending clinical courses for medical students, where they cluttered up the amphitheater and generally inconvenienced the doctors and doctors-to-be. Cornet argued that professional instruction should take place "*en famille*" (by which he meant, ironically, "only among men"), "and not in front of society ladies whose role is limited to be or become a docile auxiliary of every physician in his daily practice."[41] Parisian Dr. Chancel, speaking for his fifty colleagues in the Société Médicale des Gobelins, complained that the courses offered in the Red Cross schools "teach the complete minor surgery to a multitude of ladies." Rather than confining themselves to legitimate nursing duties, "these amateur-nurses give massages, shots, administer electricity . . . with the authorization of the institutional doctors. It is," Chancel noted, "a serious abuse that grows daily."[42] Several other physicians singled out the courses offered by the Union des Femmes de France as violating the 1892 law against the illegal practice of medicine. One went so far as to demand "the restriction of these classes and the suppression of the diplomas."[43]

But the greatest professional threat posed by the Red Cross was not excessive ambition or intrusions in medical school amphitheaters, but the proliferation of Red Cross dispensaries. Much to the distress of the medical profession, these free clinics—there were 51 in Paris by July 1910—were beginning to attract patients not only from the poorest sectors of the population (for which they were intended), but from the working class which furnished a significant percentage of the doctors' clientèle. In January 1910, the issue came up before the Parisian General Council of the Sociétés Médicales d'Arrondissement. "The patient has abandoned the doctor who has cared for him so often for many years and whom he should regard most highly," a doctor from the XIIIth *arrondissement* lamented. Instead, the patient has "rushed to these free consultations." The clientèle of the doctors in that district had, as a result of the clinics, dropped by at least a quarter. With not a little righteous indignation, the doctor insisted that the dispensaries confine their services "to the poor and indigent and leave all other patients to the physicians who have completed long courses of study and who pay a patent and who . . . ask only to be allowed to earn an honest living by working." The doctor voiced particular concern that the dispensaries not steal away working-class victims of occupational accidents whose medical bills were paid by employers or insurance companies.[44] The societies of the Red Cross had overstepped their bounds with respect to doctors and trained nurses alike. With few individual exceptions, both trained nurses and doctors agreed that the nursing services provided by the Red Cross volunteers should be limited to times of war.[45]

In addition to professional concerns, detractors pointed out the inherent unsuitability of the upper-class feminine character and way of life to the nursing profession. Critics assumed that volunteers were, in the words of one Red Cross nursing student, "society ladies who come over there to distract themselves with a new disguise, to amuse themselves . . . with toys of polished steel and glass; to artfully apply compresses, . . . bandages on undoubtedly selected wounds that did not risk offending delicate persons."[46] Lande sarcastically reminded the Red Cross ladies that "one cannot apply dressings with fingers weighted down with rings," and that the nursing uniform "does not include lace scarves or ruffles." Cosmetics and perfume, he added, are "useless and consequently dangerous" for the nurse.[47]

Lande and his fellow reformers feared that the privileged status conferred on these women by the state legitimized a new and powerful image of the nurse. If the struggle to free nursing from its congregational identity began in the 1880s, and efforts to elevate the occupation out of its servant-class status and into the realm of middle-class careers began at the turn of the century, then the battle to wrest the image of the nurse from the grip of the upper-class Red Cross "lady-volunteers" was engaged in 1908.

When hostilities broke out in Europe in the summer of 1914, the French Service de Santé Militaire—the division of the Ministry of War responsible for health services—found itself severely underequipped for a long conflict with high casualties. On August 1, 1914, fewer than 11,000 men were actively serving as nurses in the regular French army.[48] The problem of a numerically insufficient nursing corps was compounded by the already poor and rapidly sinking professional reputation of the existing staff. The recruitment problems of the turn of the century that had served as an incentive for the introduction of female lay nurses now bore bitter fruit in the form of an inadequate military nursing corps. Male nurses were often drawn from the ranks of those deemed physically, mentally, or behaviorally unsuited for other military functions. One doctor stationed in a military hospital observed during the war that his nursing staff consisted exclusively of a *personnel de fortune,* men who "never served in the army and the majority absolute strangers to the nursing profession."[49] Similarly, a volunteer nurse from England wrote that in the civilian and military *hôpital-mixte* in the Ariège, where she was stationed, the *infirmiers* "consisted, for the most part, of the wrecks of the army, of those who were physically unfit for service, and of the men who rather than go to the front would do anything, even nurse the sick and wounded, if that would save them from it."[50] Alfred Mignon, a wartime medical inspector-general, recalled that "our nursing personnel was professional only in name. The *service de santé* forgot to build a healthy and robust health corps . . . It had imagined . . . that a nurse (*infirmier*) could be created without apprenticeship by the simple decision of the recruitment commander."[51]

The beginning of the war exacerbated the recruitment problem by drafting the most able-bodied of the male nurses from both military and civilian hospitals into combat troops. By the fall of 1914, Troussaint, the director of the Service de Santé Militaire, was already engaged in what would become a long-term battle with the army general command to prevent the wholesale drafting of experienced male nurses into the infantry. The national nursing union, the Fédération des Services de Santé, voiced its outrage that authorities had no regard for the skills and experience of male nurses who had served for years in civilian hospitals before the war. These professionals, the syndicate leaders argued in 1916, "are everywhere, except where their skills dictate they should be." The military authorities retained in the hospitals and ambulances only "carpenters, notary clerks, masons, farmers, clergymen in particular, and few or no nurses."[52] Troussaint's repeated requests that the Service de Santé alone should decide which personnel were necessary for the functioning of the military hospitals went largely unheeded.[53]

As the war dragged on, the men who did end up serving as *infirmiers militaires* were increasingly likely to be inexperienced and untrained. The physician-legislator Amédée Peyroux, speaking before the Chamber of Deputies in August 1915, blamed the Minister of War for failing to build an authentically professional military nursing corps. "The male nurses know everything except their job," he argued. Their ranks were made up of "clergymen, journalists, lawyers, servants; in short, all kinds except military nurses.[54] A British nurse, stationed in France in 1915, reported that the *infirmiers* in the military hospital where she worked "forgot to wash their hands, except after a dressing, would feel if the boiled water were hot with their dirty fingers and rummaged indiscriminately in the sterilized gauze or wool box, leave dirty dressings lying about on a bed or the floor, or a table, and never . . . cleaned up a basin they had used."[55]

Even before the war actually began, it had become apparent that wartime health services could not function without the addition of large numbers of women. Yet beyond the introduction of the 96 professional lay nurses who had won their positions through national competition, the government had no plan for the training and integration of female nurses. Instead, the Ministry of War, by a decree promulgated on May 2, 1913, granted the French Red Cross the exclusive right to recruit and provide suitable personnel to treat sick and wounded soldiers during times of war. Doctors, surgeons, nurses, orderlies, and general services workers (cooks and laundry workers, for example) not directly engaged by the military were required to affiliate with one of the three Red Cross societies in order to serve in a military or auxiliary hospital. (The latter institutions were owned and organized by the different societies.) Only the approximately 10,000 members of religious congregations who served from the beginning of the war in auxiliary military hospitals of all sorts were exempt from this requirement.[56] All health-care facilities serving the military—including those that were established, supplied, and staffed by the French Red Cross itself—were explicitly and directly under the authority of the Service de Santé of the Ministry of War, a situation that would become a source of considerable friction by 1916.[57]

From the beginning of the war, the term *infirmière militaire* was virtually synonymous in the public and official mind with the Red Cross volunteers.[58] Tens of thousands of women flocked to the local branches of the three societies to volunteer their services. According to the Red Cross organizations themselves, the SSBM alone furnished somewhere between 14,000 and 17,000 nurses and nurses' aides, and the UFF, the second largest of the three Red Cross societies, supplied approximately 12,000 on the day that hostilities began.[59] Thousands more enrolled in classes that would earn them the diploma or certificate required of lay personnel providing direct patient care in any military hospital or ambulance.[60] In the first few weeks of the war, the UFF issued 4,000 certificates of *aides-auxiliaires de guerre* and 790 nursing certificates and diplomas. By December 1915, the society had delivered over 10,000 degrees of various kinds, all entitling recipients to serve in military medical facilities. The ADF, the smallest of the organizations, had issued between 6,000 and 7,000 nursing diplomas by January 1, 1916, and the SSBM distributed more than 15,000 nursing degrees in addition to 11,480 auxiliary certificates over the same time period.[61]

Observers spoke of a sea of Red Cross uniforms swarming through the streets of the nation's cities, a "veritable vertigo of charity and abnegation."[62] As one writer observed in 1916, "In the first moments of enthusiasm, . . . one can say that from one end of France to the other, all women discovered in themselves an aptitude for nursing."[63] "Mothers, wives, daughters, sisters of mobilized men were overcome with a *superbe élan* to serve their country."[64] The crush of volunteers was so great during the early weeks of the war that the editors of *La France de Bordeaux et du Sud-Ouest* urged all those who did not already hold medical degrees or nursing diplomas not to apply for military service, as they would "only create the most deplorable congestion, to the great detriment of the wounded soldiers." Sporting a Red Cross nurse's uniform became so fashionable in the early months of the war that the French Ministry of War was compelled to issue regulations in March 1915 stipulating that only accredited nurses who were bona fide members of one of the three Red Cross societies were permitted to wear the organization's dress and insignia.[65]

The sudden presence of thousands of enthusiastic but unevenly trained women in the hospital wards elicited several types of responses. Most prevalent was unstinting praise for these heroic, patriotic, selfless women who served as the perfect complement to the heroic warrior.[66] The sentimental poem entitled "L'Infirmière," which appeared in a pamphlet issued by the SSBM in 1918, closed with a typical comparison between the sacrifice of the soldier and that of the nurse. Once victory has been achieved, the poet wrote, "Our soldiers, heroes of the war," will stand "reunited," close to "the nurses, / Their humble sisters of charity."[67] The female nurse and the male combatant represented the two faces of patriotic duty: that of masculine heroism defined by the heroic act, and that of feminine charity, epitomized by humble service and self-abnegation. Medical inspector-general Alfred Mignon rhapsodized that "the beautiful blood of France filled the heart of our valiant assistants (*collaboratrices*) with the same ardor that flowed in the veins of our immortal soldiers."[68] Likewise, a contributor to *Le Flambeau* reasoned that "the maternal heart of women, *by kindness*" perfectly complements "*the valor*" of male patriotism (original emphasis).[69]

In another common formulation, admirers described the Red Cross volunteers simultaneously as heroines, saints, and, especially, mothers. Speaking before the general assembly of the SSBM in 1914, Henry Lavédan of the Académie Française stated "that the services rendered by the nurse are the most difficult and the greatest. . . . All her thoughts, all her noble desires, all her gestures and her intelligence and her kindness will come to be worked on the weakness and sadness of the soldier . . . The nurse . . . will always have, in the rapt and troubled gaze of the wounded, the stature and allure of a mother."[70] Army chaplain Félix Klein observed in 1915 how the nurse, "mother-like, . . . washes and combs her patient, while questioning him about his night of pain."[71] The nurse Germaine J. Legrix recalled the "unforgettable . . . joy of the wounded at our arrival. . . . They told us, some with tears in their eyes, that it was as if they saw their mothers and sisters coming."[72] Even a German superior officer, who was cared for by French Red Cross nurses in Noyon, was quoted thanking the French nurses who had "bolstered my courage and replaced my dear wife at my bedside."[73]

Numerous accounts also cast the nurse as a symbol of the nation itself, serving to remind the fallen soldier of everything he was fighting for. In an inspirational pamphlet addressed to the volunteers, Monseigneur Touchet, Bishop of Orléans, told the nurses that by the soldiers' "side, you are the true presence of the succoring *Patrie*."[74] The reams of sentimental poetry inspired by the legions of female volunteer nurses frequently echoed this theme. One particularly overwrought elegy informed the Red Cross nurses that "the Soldier finds in you his true treasure of war / France, its jewel of peace."[75]

Despite the heavy emphasis on feminine patriotism, the devotional dimension of wartime nursing was never far beneath the surface of descriptions of women's volunteer efforts. Far from contradicting the patriotic function of nursing work, the religious character ascribed to women's volunteer efforts complemented, even enhanced, their patriotic nature. Andrée d'Alix, a prominent spokeswoman for the conservative Catholic group, L'Action Sociale de la Femme, described the Red Cross as a "sacred militia" for which prospective nurses undergo "a moral preparation, a novitiate of charity which will exalt and strengthen them through its view of suffering itself."[76] A writer for the popular *L'Illustration* noted approvingly that the "somewhat monkish" Red Cross uniform "communicates to those who wear it the fever of devotion and charitable passion of the nuns whom they resemble."[77] In a similar vein, Jules Combarieu, author of *Les Jeunes Filles françaises et la guerre,* praised "that blue and white uniform which, with its insignias of devotion, seems to add the mysticism of the religious habit and constitutes, during wartime, women's supreme elegance!"[78] For the most pious among the Red Cross volunteers, nurses could even serve as stand-ins for those who cared for Christ in his dying moments. An official Red Cross "Prayer of the Lady Nurses of France" beseeched Jesus Christ that in the event that a soldier dies of his wounds, the nurse be able to "replace, with dignity, those holy women who received your inanimate body, and to whom it was granted to wash with their hands your five wounds."[79]

But the same feminine qualities that drew rhapsodic praise from the likes of the Bishop of Orléans, the popular press, and the Red Cross societies themselves were, to some military doctors, dangerous elements in the military hospital ward. Troussaint, director of the Service de Santé Militaire during the first years of the war, estimated that "the great majority of the medical corps" feared the transformation of venerable, feminine "sentiments of charity" into "an emotional pity whose manifestations could have an unfortunate effect on the morale of the wounded." One doctor claimed that the presence of auxiliary (Red Cross) women "had a bad effect on discipline [and] on the regularity of treatments." In particular, he noted, the women constituted "a softening influence" injected between the "courage" of the soldiers and the "will of the doctor." The "deplorable result" was nothing less than the possible loss, on the part of soldier and doctor alike, of the "precise feeling for their duty." Far from bringing joy, hope, and comfort to the wounded men, women auxiliaries threatened to feminize the military hospital and thereby break the ties that bound doctor and soldier in an exclusively masculine world of courage, honor, and duty. In this formulation, the military hospital constituted a realm that women could not enter without disturbing.[80]

While assertions that women simply did not belong at the bedside of a fallen combatant appear infrequently in the historical record, far more common were doubts about the new nurses' competence and criticism of the length and content of their training. Although the Red Cross organizations had united under a central coordinating committee in 1907, by the time the war started they still had no uniform standards for training or requirements leading to degrees.[81] The SSBM, for example, issued a *diplôme simple* to students who completed a two-month-long course of study that included classes and *stages* in hospital wards. To receive a *diplôme de guerre*, the aspiring nurse had to serve a six-month-long *stage* in a hospital and pass an exam based on theoretical material presented in the classroom. The UFF, by contrast, gave out five different certificates and diplomas, with training requirements ranging from three months of classroom work to six months of theoretical and on-the-ward training.[82] Historian Françoise Thébaud estimates that of the approximately 70,000 female benevolent workers attached to the Service de Santé by 1918, almost all held nursing diplomas of one sort or another.[83]

What kind of training or experience those degrees represented remained, at best, questionable, especially in the minds of those who had struggled to gain acceptance for nursing as a highly skilled profession and vocation. To them, the eagerness with which the Red Cross societies distributed nursing credentials and the willingness of the public and the government alike to recognize—even venerate—those degrees were alarming trends. The Swiss doctor and nursing school director Charles Krafft blamed the International Red Cross Society for failing to define a set of professional qualifications and proficiency standards for the female wartime nursing corps of the different national Red Cross organizations. "The privilege of being a member of a Red Cross Society," he wrote in a 1915 pamphlet, "should not be accorded, as it is now-a-days, to all and sundry who have followed a short course of lectures on amateur nursing."[84] The expansion of the title "*infirmière*" to incorporate all women, regardless of training and experience, implied a devaluation of the skill and commitment of the professional practitioner. The war had made "a travesty" out of nursing, a British nurse stationed in Paris in 1914 lamented. "The only person who is resented on all sides is the thoroughly trained, skilled hospital nurse, who knows her work." Though he did not single out the French case, Krafft likewise deplored the "invasion of the nursing ranks by ladies who have taken short courses of lectures on nursing." The privileged position granted to these women constituted "an injustice to professional nurses."[85]

Reports of the incompetence of the Red Cross volunteers proliferated during the early years of the war. The *British Journal of Nursing*, which regularly recounted the experiences of English nurses working in French hospitals, offered numerous harsh assessments of the "lady nurses." "It has been impossible to organize nursing in a large institution [in France], with probably 120 untrained helpers, who insisted on doing dressings . . . feeding the patients with delicacies, and then gazing with amazement at our attempt to make beds and keep things clean," one English nurse wrote. Another complained that in the hospital where she had been stationed in the north of France, "about 200 ladies (untrained, of course)" insisted upon "doing the dressings of the most serious kind." The more experienced religious sisters were forced "to give way to the Dames de France." Yet another, writing from Paris, called the volunteers an "army of masqueraders" who used "every means in their power to keep the professional woman from coming near the wounded."[86] Mabel T. Boardman, chairman of the National Relief Board of the American Red Cross, noted in 1915 that "in France professional trained nursing hardly exists. . . . To make up for this deficiency many of the women of France have taken a few weeks' course with hospital practice to prepare themselves for their country's call."[87] The purported ignorance of volunteer nurses even found its way into popular French magazines, which frequently mocked the starry-eyed young women. For example, a cartoon entitled "The Misunderstanding" published in *Le Flambeau* in 1915, showed a *docteur-majeur* examining a soldier's knee while a young Red Cross nurse looks on. "This has a large abcess," observes the doctor, "How annoying . . . One must open the eyes! (*Faut ouvrir l'oeil!*). The nurse replies, astonished, "Heavens! Doctor . . . the eyes!!!"[88]

The result of haphazard training, Charles Krafft noted, was that the sick and wounded soldiers were "much less well tended than they should have been." As tragic proof, he added, one had only to note "the immense and unforeseen number of avoidably septic cases." By the summer of 1918, Anna Hamilton, who harbored a longstanding aversion to the *dames-infirmières*, reported that "all those Red Cross amateur people," instead of providing much needed assistance for the overcrowded wards of the Maison de Santé Protestante, "have been a great trial," rendering it impossible for Hamilton to have any "real holidays" since the beginning of hostilities. "When the war broke out," she recalled in 1920, "our hospital was crowded by amateur Red Cross ladies and I had a most awful time." The volunteers were "very unruly as to hours on or off duty, *refusing* to do night duty more than *one* night at a time and not more often than *once* a week!" (original emphasis).[89]

Physicians and surgeons continued to complain, as they had before the war, about the Red Cross volunteers' penchant for treading on their professional turf. A "doctoresse," writing in 1916, noted her colleagues' pervasive fear of the "semi-bluestockings of medicine." When recruiting volunteer nurses, some ambulance teams went so far as to take as their watchword, "Especially no women with diplomas!" The military doctor Tridon reminded UFF nursing students in 1918 never to alter or interpret a doctor's instructions, and to "confine yourself to your own beautiful and immense role and do not think that you aggrandize yourselves by encroaching on the doctors." It was the physician's responsibility to "operate, bandage, prescribe"; the nurse was there to "assure [his] success."[90] The doctors could not allow the presence of women whose social-class background was comparable—at times even superior—to their own, to upset the gender-based system of professional authority in the military hospital.

Yet if it is true that many volunteers rushed to the cause with little more than a few months of instruction, other Red Cross nurses had substantial training and years of experience. A number of them had served in Morocco in 1907 and 1911 and aided Parisian flood victims in 1910. Those who joined the Red Cross in the patriotic tidal wave that swept the nation in the aftermath of the first Moroccan crisis often went on to spend at least two years on a hospital ward or in a dispensary. Charlotte Maitre, an *infirmière-major* of the ADF and designated a Knight of the Legion of Honor in 1917, had received a nursing diploma from the Ecole Française des Infirmières de Paris before leaving for the front. In addition to working in the wards in hospitals in Louhans and Lyons, she directed the nursing staff at the military Val-de-Grâce Hospital and served as an inspector for the Service de Santé.[91] The employment record of SSBM nurse Mademoiselle Juliard, the only one of its kind to survive in the Red Cross archives, reveals an uninterrupted career dating from 1905 through 1919. Her training included more than two years assisting doctors in the Paris Hôtel-Dieu. By 1909 she had won accolades from numerous physicians and received a Diplôme supérieur and Diplôme d'administration des hôpitaux militaires. In 1910 she was hired by the Service de Santé as a nurse in Val-de-Grâce Hospital, and after two months she was sent to Morocco, where she remained until June of 1914. Over the next five years Juliard served in at least nine different military hospitals, mostly in operating rooms in evacuation hospitals, ambulances, and *auto-chirurgicales* near or at the front, always winning the highest praise from the doctors with whom she worked. In 1922 she received her State Diploma "by equivalence," in recognition of her 16-year-long apprenticeship.[92]

While the careers of Maitre and Juliard were probably not representative of most Red Cross nurses, it is also clear that they were not completely isolated examples. Popular journals and official Red Cross publications recounted the heroic tales of dozens of volunteers who served through the entire war in various nursing capacities. Expressing the sentiment of many contemporary observers, the army chaplain Félix Klein noted that many nurses "have taken no rest since the opening of the hospital, and when one remembers that most of them are people of Society, accustomed to an idle life, one is struck with admiration for such self-sacrifice."[93] If their formal training remained questionable, then surely their years of wartime duty had dispelled suspicions that they had joined the Red Cross for amusement.

Their growing record of achievement notwithstanding, the large numbers of affluent women in military hospitals and other facilities raised questions about the appropriate class status of the nurse. The matter had come up earlier in the century, first in the context of Anna Hamilton's efforts to attract middle-class women to the profession, and later with the admission of Red Cross "ladies" into the military hospital wards in 1908. At issue during the war was whether middle- and upper-class women who did not have to work for wages were capable of performing the strenuous, unglamorous, and frequently tedious work of hospital nursing. Would they, in other words, be able to subordinate their civilian social identity to the exigencies of the wartime medical ward, where the patients were classed according to the severity of their illness or injury and their caregivers by the level of their medical expertise?

Many observers answered that question in the negative, as they had in 1908, castigating the women for dressing and behaving in a manner that stressed the frivolous and coquettish aspects of femininity rather than its modesty, devotion, and compassion.[94] One British nurse who served in France described a hospital of 500 patients as reminding her of "opera bouffe." Everywhere, she wrote, one found "ladies dressed in the height of fashion, . . . some with slit skirts, silk stockings, high heels on dainty shoes, diamonds and pearls on necks, wrists and fingers." Ostentatious displays of wealth and social status could only promote discord within the ranks of the nurses. Mlle. Génin, *directrice* of the flagship Hôpital-Ecole of the SSBM in Paris, reminded the Red Cross nurses that, like soldiers whose civilian social status disappeared beneath the military uniform, nurses must forget all class hierarchy. "As soon as you don the nurse's blouse, you are all equal."[95]

Women who flaunted their affluence also risked distancing themselves from their patients. Dr. Tridon, a Red Cross doctor, warned students and nurses at a UFF nursing school in Amiens against coquetry of all kinds. Explicitly discouraging "too much elegance" and the wearing of jewelry, the physician urged the women to minimize the obvious signs of class difference between the volunteer "lady-nurses" and their patients. "Remember," he advised, "that your patients are above all farmers, workers, simple men, unaccustomed to the display of feminine graces." Nurses should take pains not to irritate the men by "showing yourselves to be very different from their mothers and wives, field or factory workers."[96]

Although wealthy and prominent women tended to dominate press coverage of the nurses' experiences, not all Red Cross nurses came from the upper classes. For example, in 1915 Le Flambeau ran an intriguing article about a group of garment workers who, under the leadership of the composer Gustave Charpentier, had formed a singing ensemble. When the war broke out, the women traded their music lessons for nursing training, and by the fall of 1915 were serving in four different hospitals. While the musical angle and the women's attachment to the prominent composer made them particularly newsworthy, the phenomenon of garment workers volunteering for nursing duty was clearly unusual enough to merit notice in and of itself.[97]

Despite their many critics, the Red Cross volunteers retained the support of state officials and much of the medical corps. Their positive opinions may well have been influenced by their awareness of the value of currying favor with the "lady volunteers." Many Red Cross volunteers had substantial financial resources and were eager to put that money to patriotic use. New members of the societies had to contribute upwards of 600FF to their chosen organization to cover the "right of membership, dues, and uniforms." Annual dues amounted to 30FF.[98] By the time of the armistice, Red Cross financial contributions to the war effort exceeded half a billion francs, or more than twenty percent of the total costs of the Service de Santé.[99] The wealthiest and most generous contributors funded entire hospitals, sometimes situated in their private châteaux, which they often demanded to direct. Mlle. de Baye, for example, purchased surgical equipment and a team of fourteen nurses, which she offered to put at the disposal of the Service de Santé on the condition that she hold the title of surintendante. De Baye obtained her first post through the direct intervention of General Pétain himself (a position from which she was eventually dismissed for abuse of authority).[100] In another example, chaplain Félix Klein praised Mme. G., the wife of a Corneuve manufacturer, who, "not content with keeping the wives and children of her husband's employees during the War, . . . undertakes the expenses of the hospital," which she also directed.[101] In still another instance, an English nurse described a young woman "with heaps of money" who had become "quite the *Directrice*" of her own hospital. "She has never been trained for a day, but wears full nursing canonicals, and just provides everything up-to-date for treatment that the doctors need, so is highly regarded." Another complained that there had been a constant turnover in matrons and nurses in her hospital, "simply because the laywomen who get the money from the public to keep it going will interfere with things they know nothing about . . . always treading on professional toes."[102] Even the religious congregations were often in a position to donate their orphanages, convalescent institutions, and homes for the elderly to the cause. As a result, a significant number of the auxiliary medical facilities were staffed exclusively or predominantly by the congregations.

Career nurses had no comparable assets and feared that their hard-won qualifications paled beside the high profile of the Red Cross volunteers. Not only did the former lack the attractive power of money, but their limited numbers and tendency to remain in civilian hospitals (many of which were requisitioned in whole or in part for military use) translated into professional invisibility. Although some nurses who had served in hospitals before the war left their positions to join Red Cross units closer to the action, most could not afford to forfeit their salaries for volunteer work. Many therefore remained at less "glamorous" posts in the cities and towns, where their skills were desperately needed to treat serious injuries and especially the rapidly growing numbers of typhoid, tuberculosis, and influenza cases.[103]

Some nurses and nursing reformers viewed the war as an opportunity to prove the value of the trained professional. Anna Hamilton admitted that "at first it seemed as if our professional nurses were going to be put aside [for] not belonging to the Red Cross Societies." But, she stated in 1917, the highly trained students of the Maison de Santé Protestante had never been more useful than since the beginning of the war. "Our nurses are in great demand and everywhere are so much appreciated." This, she fervently hoped, would translate into heightened regard for "the professional nurse truly deserving of the name so that one of the benefits of this sad war will be to dispel the prejudice of which they [sic] are the object."[104]

Given the MSP's modest size, its contributions to the war effort were indeed impressive. Designated by the military in 1914 as Auxiliary Hospital No. 2, the MSP received many of the army's most serious cases. By the time the auxiliary facility was closed in January 1919, MSP nurses had treated 1,146 wounded soldiers. As of August 1916, thirty-seven MSP graduates had served in twenty-three different military hospitals or *hôpitaux-mixtes* (serving both civilian and military patients) from Cannes to Besançon to Saintes to Pau. In addition, 65 students joined 11 auxiliary hospitals run by the various Red Cross societies, including institutions in Paris, Rouen, Montpellier, and Nancy, and several took posts with the Italian and Belgian Red Cross organizations. Most of these women received no pay, and only some were given food and housing. Hamilton noted proudly that MSP nurses held 58 positions of authority, ranging from *directrice* to *infirmière-major* (nursing team leader) and *chef de salle* (ward head). Most, however, accepted posts as "*simples gardes-malades*" tendering direct patient care in the wards.[105]

Nursing leaders and doctors alike praised the Bordeaux graduates for their respect for professional boundaries and hierarchy within the hospitals. The *British Journal of Nursing* observed approvingly that at the MSP, unlike the Red Cross schools, "emphasis is laid on the fact that the work of nurses is primarily to care for the sick and not to be inferior doctors." Graduate nurses were told "to leave the theatres [of operations] and dressing-rooms to the care of students of medicine" and confine themselves to the wards, where they had the best chance of proving themselves "the most valued assistants to the medical profession."[106] Real professional nurses knew their proper place; excessive ambition was the hallmark of the amateur.

Although advocates of professional nursing worried that the image of the untrained volunteer had obliterated that of the trained nurse, a few signs emerged during the war suggesting that the distinction between amateur and professional had not completely evaporated. True, the Service de Santé had delegated to the Red Cross the task of training and recruiting the majority of the female nursing staff for the war. But within months of the opening of hostilities, the Ministry of War hired 300 professional nurses from the British Commonwealth (including English, Irish, Scottish, and Canadian women) to augment the French staff. Members of this French Flag Nursing Corps (FFNC) served under the direct authority of the Ministry of War and drew salaries identical to those received by French military nurses. Like the graduates of the MSP, the women of the FFNC were often appointed to supervisory positions and, in several instances, were entrusted with the responsibility of organizing the entire nursing staff of a hospital. The new 700-bed military hospital in Talence near Bordeaux, for example, was staffed entirely by FFNC members until 1917, when Americans assumed control of the institution.[107]

The French Flag Nursing Corps, along with the hundreds of foreigners from neutral and allied countries who volunteered to serve as nurses in France, provided crucial support for the severely strained Service de Santé Militaire. In hiring the FFNC nurses, the Ministry of War implicitly acknowledged the value of professional nurses: all had completed at least three years of formal training, spoke fluent French, and most had several years of experience working in a hospital. In a parliamentary session in August 1915, Deputy Amédée Peyroux accused Service de Santé Director Troussaint of using the British nurses to compensate for the inadequacies of the French nursing corps. Troussaint could hardly have denied the charge given the flood of volunteers, both French and foreign, who crowded hospital wards in the early months of the war. While there was clearly no need simply for more bodies, competent, experienced professionals remained at a premium. Aware that the FFNC women had expertise that most of their French counterparts lacked, the director of the Service de Santé even went so far as to send nurses, midwives, and Red Cross volunteers to attend classes on "the theory and practice of nursing" offered by the FFNC matron of the Talence Hospital.[108]

The British nurses, for their part, thought of themselves not just as contributors to the war effort of their political ally, but also as missionaries for "the science and practice of nursing à l'Anglaise." When the first group of British nurses arrived in France in November 1914, the Scottish director of the FFNC, Grace Ellison, observed that each supervising doctor was issued a "typed definition of what a nurse was," which explained her "social position" and the meaning of her diploma. "No one had the least idea of what a British trained nurse was," she lamented. One British nurse complained that among the most difficult aspects of organizing patient care in a French military hospital was getting "the medical men to realise the meaning of 'certificated' nurses and to recognise our nursing powers." In her experience, doctors often preferred men "by trade anything" over a highly competent *diplomée*.[109]

Less than four months later, Ellison reported that the FFNC nurses had already won converts among the nurses and doctors alike. "Many French ladies are anxious to work under the English Sisters and learn their nursing methods," she wrote in July of 1915.[110] Dr. R. Mougeot, *médecin-major* and mayor of St. Dizier in the Haute-Marne, conceded that "from the technical point of view it would be impossible not to appreciate them." The French doctors in Rouen's Hôtel-Dieu praised the British unit stationed there as "quick, clean, clever, tactful, and thoroughly reliable," and insisted that upon their transfer to Bordeaux, they be replaced by other English nurses. At the war's end, a Paris official of the Service de Santé credited FFNC members with being "the most satisfactory of all the nurses—English, French, or American—who have worked under its formation." Should "any of them care to remain on, after the signing of peace," he added, "we shall be only too pleased to place them in their various formations."[111] Few, if any, British nurses accepted the invitation, but the offer itself suggests that the French Ministry of War was interested in improving the standards of French nursing.

All the same, the Service de Santé had yet to prove its commitment to establishing formal guidelines for the training of French military nurses. The creation in 1916 of the state-sponsored Hôpital-Ecole Edith Cavell for the training of military nurses replicated the problems of the Red Cross schools by requiring only three months of training. FFNC director Grace Ellison, who drew up the initial plans for the school in 1915, had originally intended it to be run entirely by English nurses and graduates of the MSP. Ellison later resigned from the organizing committee, after the private Parisian organization, the Association pour le Développement de l'Assistance aux Malades, in conjunction with the Service de Santé, insisted on a Paris-based faculty and a drastically reduced training period. Sharing Ellison's disappointment in the modified standards of the new program, Anna Hamilton argued that the Association promoted the idea of nursing as a "society fad" and that the Edith Cavell School was "an insult to the name of that splendid nurse."[112]

The Service de Santé's refusal to acknowledge the importance of a lengthy and thorough instructional period was largely the product of necessity. By 1916, the surfeit of nurses that had characterized the first year of the war had evaporated. The ranks of Red Cross volunteers had thinned as the early enthusiasm for the ever-lengthening war waned; above all, many women, especially those who had lost their husbands either permanently or temporarily to the war, could not afford to work indefinitely without a living wage. The new director of the Service de Santé, Justin Godart, needed replacements quickly; he could not afford to wait a year or even six months while volunteers received proper training.[113]

A similar pragmatism motivated the Service de Santé to initiate the only significant reform in the organization of military nursing during the war: the recruitment, in March 1916, of a corps of temporary, government-paid nurses. The measure called on any French woman who was at least 21 years old, in good health, and "possessing the requisite knowledge to be of use to the Service de Santé" to commit herself to serve in the nation's military hospitals for the duration of the war plus six months after the armistice.[114] The announcement of the new policy met with sharp opposition from the Red Cross societies, which, for the first time since the war began, had to compete with the government for nursing recruits. They feared primarily that the financial incentives offered by the government would lure away both new volunteers and experienced workers.[115]

Those apprehensions were not without foundation, as many capable women saw in the new program a much-needed means of earning a living, and in some cases, supporting a family. The prefecture of the Gironde, for example, received a flurry of letters from women with midwifery diplomas requesting paid employment as temporary war nurses. In one case, a woman who held a second-class midwifery diploma entitling her to practice only in the department of the Charente-Inferior, found herself living with relatives in Deux-Sèvres, where she was not permitted to work as a midwife. She eventually received an appointment in a Bordeaux military hospital. Similarly, Marie Louise-Marguerite Vuillet, who had earned her second-class midwifery diploma from the Académie d'Accouchement in Besançon, explained that she had been forced to leave her job in Doubs (the only department where her diploma authorized her to practice) to join her husband, who had just been demobilized and sent to Saint-André de Cubzac near Bordeaux to improve his "delicate" health. With two young children at home, she could not survive on her husband's salary and begged for a position as a temporary nurse in a Bordeaux hospital. In another instance, Mlle. Gabrielle Lacaze, who had already served for three months as a benevolent nurse in the contagious diseases ward of a Bordeaux hospital, requested a paid position as *infirmière militaire* in "any health facility or hospital whatsoever." The director of Service de Santé appointed her "infirmière titulaire de 3me classe" three months later. The Red Cross tried to counter the government's move by granting small indemnities to cover its nurses' expenses, but it still lost significant numbers of volunteers.[116]

The new policy amounted to a sharp slap in the face for the Red Cross, and their supporters responded in kind. The *Revue hebdomadaire* chastised the Service de Santé for alienating the wealthy societies, thereby forfeiting "so casually . . . so many material and moral resources," and for provoking what amounted to "a second war," this one between the Service de Santé and the Red Cross. Tensions mounted in the ensuing months over government policies that seemed to favor nurses employed directly by the Service de Santé over their Red Cross counterparts. In October 1916, the Service de Santé forged an agreement with the railroad companies whereby half-price rail tickets were granted only to those nurses "recruited and administered by the Service de Santé" and to "benevolent nurses" (those who served without pay) not belonging to the Red Cross. The Red Cross societies also complained that the new temporary nurses received higher quality food than their Red Cross counterparts. Toward the end of the war rumors circulated in the general and medical press that the army was trying to eliminate the Red Cross completely.[117]

The final insult came in February 1917, when the director of the Service de Santé suggested a number of changes in the 1913 policy governing the relationship between the Red Cross and the government. Included among the proposed alterations was the creation of a disciplinary council, controlled by the Service de Santé, which would regulate the behavior of all voluntary medical and nursing personnel. The measure elicited a furious response from Louis Renault, president of the SSBM, who deplored the "attack on the . . . autonomy of the societies."[118] The Service de Santé eventually withdrew the proposal, after the Red Cross agreed to set up its own internally administered disciplinary council.

Red Cross leaders were particularly enraged by the absence of any standards of training for the temporary nurses. Dr. P. Bouloumié, secretary general of the UFF, noted accurately that only as a last requirement (and then only "should the occasion arise") did the new "Instruction" ask applicants to furnish diplomas or certificates testifying to their training and experience. Even the *American Journal of Nursing*, certainly no supporter of the French Red Cross nurses, stated that the "moral and educational standards [of the temporary corps] were so low as to be positively non-existent." The very criticism that had so frequently been lodged against the

Red Cross societies now became their own weapon against the Service de Santé.[119]

While the creation of the corps of temporary nurses hardly represented a move toward professionalization, it did broach the crucial issue of whether wartime nursing should be considered direct paid service to the state, or a particular form of uncompensated feminine patriotic duty. Despite the contemporary popularity of such slogans as "men to the front, women to the hospitals," feminine military nursing remained more closely analogous to patriotic motherhood than to male soldiering. As Margaret Darrow has written, "All agreed that volunteer nursing was personal, rather than abstract national service, that while the soldier served France, the nurse served the soldier."[120] That distinction extended to the material level. Men drafted into the army received a salary as well as food, shelter, and clothing, whereas until 1916 the Red Cross did not even supply meals for the nurses working in its own hospitals. The Ministry of War's decision to recruit and pay female nurses placed the state squarely behind the image of nursing as direct and compensated service to the state rather than as benevolent service to a voluntary organization. The decision also implied—however tentatively and inadvertently—that affluent women had no *a priori* monopoly on the romanticized image of the *dame blanche*.[121]

Yet between the salaried state worker and the skilled professional stretched a vast distance that the government's apparent rebuff of the Red Cross societies had done nothing to close. The women hired by the Service de Santé after 1917 were, after all, recruited primarily because they were women, not because they had nursing skills. By the time the guns finally fell silent in November 1918, nurses—whatever their training, expertise, or experience—had clearly won for themselves an honored, if not exactly prominent or especially enduring, place in the gallery of heroes and martyrs of the war. But it was a place occupied alike by Red Cross auxiliary-aides, experienced Red Cross nurses, members of religious congregations, wealthy benefactresses of hospitals, midwives or university students turned temporary nurses, and trained career nurses. The experience of the Great War brought lay women into military hospitals for the first time, assigning them a legitimate and specifically feminine role in what was once a strictly male domain. But the equation of "woman" and "nurse" that occurred in the process, and that lay at the root of the nurse's new-found status, undermined the project of professionalization that many reformers hoped would emerge from the war. In honoring the nurse, the public and the state honored not the skilled female expert, but the patriotic and nurturing woman; the mother, sister, and daughter who felt called to care for her family of French soldiers. In the years that followed the armistice, nursing reformers would strive to re-establish the professional boundaries that had begun to emerge in the years surrounding the turn of the century, and which the war had so effectively erased.

Nursing in Postwar France

In January 1921, the prominent social Catholic Léonie Chaptal, *directrice* of a small Parisian school for private-duty nursing, delivered a report before the Conseil Supérieur de l'Assistance Publique (CSAP) on the status of nursing in France.[1] "It is a question of a profession as old as disease," she began, "but that did not really become a profession until some years ago."[2] Chaptal did not intend to trace the evolution of nursing in France from charitable activity to skilled health care specialty; she hoped simply to convince the CSAP of the urgent need for state regulation of the profession. Citing the examples of physicians, pharmacists, and midwives, Chaptal argued that nurses too should be required to have specific credentials in order to practice their craft: "It is important for the care of the patients that the professional capability of the nurses be recognized by means of an official diploma."[3]

According to Chaptal's proposal, students aspiring to the state diploma would be required to undergo two years of training at an approved school and pass a juried, standardized exam. Accreditation of training programs would be granted by a Council for the Improvement of Nursing Schools (*Conseil de Perfectionnement des Ecoles d'Infirmières*) composed not only of doctors and administrators, but of "a number of [nursing] school directors and qualified nurses." Those seeking to specialize in the home care of tuberculosis patients (*infirmières visiteuses d'hygiène*), infants and mothers (*infirmières de puériculture*), or in becoming school nurses (*infirmières scolaires*) would undergo additional training and receive a separate diploma. In other words, the state would set the requirements for and issue diplomas that alone would authorize women to be hired as nurses.[4]

Chaptal's proposal rested on her assessment that the nursing profession had in recent years become sufficiently technically sophisticated and socially vital to warrant regulation. "The time when one could say that devotion alone sufficed to care for a patient came to an end on the day the work of Pasteur and his successors revolutionized medical science," she remarked, drawing upon a formulation that dated back to the Ministry of the Interior's turn-of-the-century circulars on the establishment of nursing schools. The danger inherent in the modern practice of nursing, coupled with its growing "public usefulness," rendered it "necessary that the State intervene and take [the profession] under its supervision, either directly or by means of an intermediary body."[5] Nursing, in Chaptal's estimation, had evolved well beyond its earlier classification as charitable duty or semi-skilled wage labor into a specialized, highly trained profession essential to the national well-being.

Efforts to establish state regulation of nursing were not a novelty of the postwar period. As early as 1908, the *Bulletin professionnel des infirmières et gardes-malades* endorsed the introduction of state exams and state licensing, arguing that formal regulation would "eliminate the crowd of know-nothings, who have more aplomb than science, who do the greatest harm to the profession."[6] That same year, the Fédération des Services de Santé de France et des Colonies (FSS) came out in favor of regulation, both as a means of promoting greater mobility among workers and of enhancing the professional value of trained lay nurses in their ongoing competition with the religious sisters.[7] Four years later, the FSS approved a motion stipulating that all the hospitals offer professional courses "with a standardized, obligatory curriculum," which would lead to "the nationalization of the [nursing] diploma."[8] Similarly, the physician and Socialist deputy from the Ardennes, Henri Doizy, proposed in 1913 that the government mandate the establishment of "schools in all the cities and hospitals to train nurses to whom would be delivered a standardized diploma that would facilitate the practice of the profession in all towns."[9] Doizy viewed the measure as particularly useful in countering recent attempts by Paris Municipal Council members to reintroduce religious congregations into the hospitals of the Assistance Publique. The Chamber of Deputies could most effectively come to the aid of the lay personnel, currently "under violent attack," by officially confirming its "unique professional competence."[10]

Chaptal's 1921 demand for state regulation did not emerge from an anticlerical agenda. To the contrary, her strong Social-Catholic beliefs rendered her rather more open to the positive contributions of religious nursing congregations than reformers like Anna Hamilton might have preferred. Her recommendations arose instead from an acute awareness of the changes in nursing that had been wrought during the war and in its immediate aftermath. Readily acknowledging that the nearly 100,000 Red Cross volunteers who had served in the nation's military hospitals and ambulances had performed a valuable service to the nation, Chaptal nonetheless maintained that the sudden and massive increase in the numbers of women calling themselves nurses had brought considerable—and potentially dangerous—disorder to the field. Dr. Gustave Dron, a CSAP member and Radical senator from the Nord, concurred wholeheartedly with Chaptal's assessment. The war certainly "caused a blossoming of nursing vocations," he noted, but the new nurses "dedicated themselves [to the profession] without the required knowledge apart from a few theoretical notions of anatomy."[11] Whereas in the chaos of wartime the mere presence of enthusiastic and well-intentioned—if undertrained—assistants in the nation's often hard-pressed medical facilities served a valuable purpose, the same did not hold true for the postwar world.

As the last of the war casualties were sent home or to permanent military or civilian hospitals in the interior, thousands of wartime nurses, whether direct employees of the Service de Santé Militaire or Red Cross volunteers, found themselves without work. Many women, especially those who were married or had financial means, returned to the *foyer*. But for the numerous temporary nurses who had relied on the salary allotted by the Service de Santé Militaire, unemployment meant the loss of vital income. As Paul Strauss, editor of the *Revue philanthropique* and future Minister of Hygiene, observed in 1921, "the harshness of the times is forcing a large number of young girls and women to find remunerative employment." Reflecting the postwar emphasis on the restabilization of society through strengthening and enlarging the family unit, the government allocated a small monthly cost-of-living stipend of 45 francs to married women (with or without children), but single women without children were left to fend for themselves. A few found permanent jobs in military hospitals, but most lacked the necessary credentials to secure those scarce positions. In June 1919, the Ministry of the Interior issued a circular to all departmental prefects asking them to notify public and private charitable establishments of the availability of "demobilized nurses, able to insure the various assistance services."[12]

In the months immediately following the war, many more attempted to ply their newly acquired trade as nurses in the civilian sector. Some managed to gain employment in municipal hospitals. The Paris Assistance Publique hospitals, for example, hired 39 war widows to serve as ward maids (*filles de services*). In 1919, the Paris Syndicat du Personnel Non-Gradé protested against the hiring of former war nurses who, the union maintained, were replacing "women with ten and fifteen years of service."[13] Other jobless nurses solicited business in the private sector, serving wealthier clients in their homes. This strategy drew strong criticism from Chaptal, who asserted that the practice of private nursing by inadequately trained women threatened both the health of the community and the integrity of the nursing profession. Too many wartime nurses "believed that they acquired the necessary knowledge in the wards that they crossed; many of them suffered, as a result of the hostilities, a severe reduction of resources; many tried to live off of this new knowledge, knowledge that was insufficient." Chaptal's own nursing school witnessed a steep decline in the number of requests for home nursing care in the immediate aftermath of the war, a trend that she attributed to the influx of nurses "more or less amateur" trying to make a living. "We did not want them," Chaptal stated bluntly, "and we did not even realize the risk that such competition could entail." The experience of 1919 vividly demonstrated to Chaptal the need for official regulation of nursing and of state support for bona fide professionals.[14]

Within a year of the conclusion of the war the problem had become less one of a surplus than of a dire shortage of nurses. The "amateurs" who had plagued Chaptal's school had faded away, and Anna Hamilton complained that the Red Cross nurses who provided much of the staff for Bordeaux's tuberculosis dispensaries had all "vanished" by summer.[15] One CSAP member, the Parisian law professor Berthélemy, predicted that "for a long time the numbers of nurses with diplomas will remain insufficient" and suggested that health-care facilities turn, at least provisionally, to those "honorable but less educated persons . . . the religious women."[16] The doctor favored the Lyons model of quasi-religious, quasi-lay nurses as a possible solution to the problem.

In Paris, the dearth of nurses soon reached crisis proportions. In June 1919, the Conseil de Surveillance de l'Assistance Publique, which oversaw the administration of all of Paris's public hospitals and hospices, reported that a minimum of 500 more *infirmières* were needed immediately to staff the city's institutions. The Conseil pointed out that the recent application of the new law on the eight-hour day to the hospitals meant that institutions that formerly had employed two work shifts now needed a third. The city's nursing schools—including both the municipal programs set up by Bourneville and the Ecole des Infirmières de l'Assistance Publique at the Salpêtrière Hospital—could furnish only a fraction of the necessary personnel. The Conseil de Surveillance regretfully now found itself "forced to call . . . on the very numerous nurses who cared for the injured and sick soldiers in the medical units."[17] The Conseil's obvious reluctance to take this step signaled not only a pervasive resistance to the application of the eight-hour day in hospitals, but an abiding mistrust of the competence of the former military nurses.[18]

In the long-term, then, the war had not spurred a noticeable expansion of nursing as a career for women, despite numerous claims to the contrary. Berthélemy noted in 1921 that when he had recently tried to convince a group of "young society girls" to take up nursing, the families had responded with incredulity: "What! Send our children into a hospital environment!" Stressing the pervasive moral laxity among nursing personnel, Berthélemy warned that upstanding young women would never consent "to commit themselves to a profession that lacks dignity in this matter." Highly regarded training programs like those run by Léonie Chaptal and by the Association pour le Développement de l'Assistance aux Malades no longer recruited sufficient numbers of students to meet the needs of the nation's health care institutions. Even Anna Hamilton complained that "since the war we have much more difficulty in getting pupils," while those who do graduate "are so much in demand and [are] offered more posts than they can hold."[19]

If the war had served to raise the status of the nursing profession, it had done so in a limited fashion and only temporarily. The prestige attached to caring for the casualties of war had been intimately tied to notions of patriotic duty, which in turn had been linked to the valorization of womanly acts of self-sacrifice. The decline in hospital nursing in the immediate postwar years was the result of the transformation of the image of nursing from voluntary act of patriotism to feminine profession. The legions of middle- and upper-class women who eagerly entered the wartime military hospitals had been attracted by a specific image of the nurse and a specific image of the hospital; both had vanished with the cessation of hostilities. Those who undertook to become paid professional nurses after the war faced a potentially lengthy training period and a long climb up the employment ladder. Perhaps even more significantly, middle-class women who decided to enter nursing professionally had to overcome not only age-old negative images of the civilian hospital—beliefs which the war had done nothing to dispel—but also culturally imbedded suspicions of women's waged labor.[20] Middle-class women, the very class of employees that the Maison de Santé Protestante and the Paris Salpêtrière school hoped to attract, could safely serve as volunteer (or even paid) nurses under the extraordinary circumstances of the war. But the postwar political and cultural ethos, promoted quite explicitly by a reactionary parliament, demanded a return to social order after the chaos of war. To many former wartime volunteer nurses, that meant a redirection of their feminine, nurturing instincts away from the nation and back to the family.[21]

Yet in some ways the postwar years constituted a golden era for nursing. With the cessation of hostilities in 1918, the French turned their attention to the daunting business of rebuilding the country. In the aftermath of more than four years of destruction, regeneration demanded far more than teams of engineers and construction workers; far more even than a massive influx of money. It required, above all, a concerted effort to revitalize a population whose low birthrate and high mortality rates (especially among newborns) stood as potent symbols of national exhaustion. Between 1850 and 1910, the French population had grown by only 3.4 million (to 39.1 million), while Germany increased its population by 25 million, to reach a total of 58.4 million (including the territories of Alsace and Lorraine acquired in 1871). The birthrate in France dipped from approximately 28 per 1,000 in 1850 to about 18 just before the war and plunged to 8 during the war itself. The comparable figures for Germany were 37 per 1,000 in 1850, 27 before the war, and 14 during the war. For seven of the years between 1890 and 1914, the French death rate exceeded the birthrate.[22]

The immediate postwar years were marked by unprecedented state interest in the physical health and well-being of French citizens. With the fighting over, health authorities in government-run and private organizations turned their full attention to such long-term public health and hygiene issues as the treatment of tuberculosis, alcoholism, and venereal disease, and the reduction of infant mortality rates. The broadest national health campaigns of the postwar years, the ones that most actively enlisted the support of female nurses, focused primarily on two large groups of victims: the poor and the tubercular (categories that became increasingly synonymous in the early twentieth century), and infants and children (especially of the poor and working class).[23] In other words, the "family" that required women's renewed attention to revitalize the nation was not just the private family of the individual woman, but the Family as a social and spiritual institution. If middle-class women would not enter the public hospitals, they could certainly enter the home, which still remained women's special domain.

To be sure, efforts to combat tuberculosis and reduce infant mortality rates predated the postwar period. In 1903, Prime Minister Emile Combes created within the Ministry of the Interior a permanent commission on the prevention of the disease. In the aftermath of defeat in the Franco-Prussian War, concerns (verging at times almost on hysteria) about the nation's stagnant population figures prompted the governments of the early Third Republic to pass significant legislation designed to improve the conditions of motherhood and infancy. The Roussel Law of 1874, for example, established a system for monitoring the safety of children put out to nurse. The Strauss Law of 1913 mandated a two-month maternity leave for mothers working in industry and commerce, and provided financial benefits for women who demonstrated their compliance with hygienic protocol. As historian Alisa Klaus has pointed out, the implementation of both of these laws relied heavily on the volunteer labor of women.[24]

In addition to these government initiatives, numerous individuals (especially wealthy philanthropists and physicians) as well as private institutions and organizations sponsored public health and social hygiene projects. In the closing years of the nineteenth century, Dr. Maurice Letulle of Lyons opened the nation's first center for the testing and treatment of tuberculosis, and in 1901, Dr. Albert Calmette established the Oeuvre Antituberculeuse du Nord.[25] The Red Cross Union des Femmes de France was instrumental in setting up special hospitals for the care of tuberculosis patients in each of the 21 military zones beginning in 1917. Similarly, the Société de Secours aux Blessés Militaires asked its local committees to put their nurses at the disposal of the departmental Commissions d'Assistance des Militaires Tuberculaires to staff special dispensaries and new treatment centers. Well before the war, efforts to improve the health of poor mothers and their children attracted particular attention from those concerned about the population crisis. The first three decades of the Third Republic witnessed the establishment of numerous private philanthropic groups geared to infant welfare, including, among many others, the Oeuvre de l'Allaitement Maternel (1876), which promoted breastfeeding among poor and working-class women; the Oeuvre Nouvelle des Crèches Parisiennes (1896), which ran nurseries for the children of working-class mothers; and the Cantines Maternelles (1905), which provided free food for nursing mothers.[26]

Nurses played a critical role in guaranteeing the success of these various public health projects. At the 1912 International Conference against Tuberculosis in Rome, Léonie Chaptal described the nurse who specialized in the disease as the single indispensable agent "if one truly wants to contain, combat, and finally, extinguish the evil." Chaptal envisioned a large corps of visiting nurses (*infirmières visiteuses*) entering working-class homes throughout the country to instruct mothers in the proper techniques for preventing infection.[27]

Until the war, the role and professional status of the visiting nurse remained a controversial issue within the medical profession. At the 1911 National Conference on Public and Private Assistance, several physicians speaking in the name of such private practitioners' associations as the Syndicat des Médecins de la Seine and the nationwide 8,000-member Concours Médical predicted that incorporating trained nurses with diplomas into the system of medical assistance to the poor would result in the widespread illegal practice of medicine. Dr. Gustave Drouineau, a member of the CSAP, proposed instead to substitute the professional *infirmière-visiteuse* with the *infirmière-ménagère* (nurse-housewife), whose only qualifications would be "an unimpeachable morality and sufficient intelligence . . . to ably assist a doctor." Needless to say, the suggestion met with harsh criticism from Anna Hamilton, who accused Drouineau of advocating the creation of a corps of "persons who were half nurses and half servants, going from house to house to offer nursing care and do housekeeping chores." In protecting its own professional interests, the medical community had cast aside an opportunity to create a real nursing specialty. Instead, once again, it relegated the nurse to the status of well-meaning charity worker or domestic servant.[28]

Despite resistance from private doctors, the idea of enlisting the skills and energy of trained women to fight the three plagues of poverty—tuberculosis, alcoholism, and infant mortality—gained momentum in the prewar years. At the 1912 International Women's Conference, the French spokesperson for the section on hygiene argued that the "creation of a

French corps of visiting nurses analogous to that of the English District Nurses" would be the most effective means of combating "the deadly ravages of tuberculosis." In February 1914, the Paris Assistance Publique administration, with the help of such prominent sponsors as Mme. la Comtesse d'Haussonville, Mme. D. Pérouse, and Mme. L. Carnot (presidents, respectively, of the Red Cross's Société de Secours aux Blessés Militaires, Union des Femmes de France, and Association des Dames Françaises) and Mme. la Marquise de Ganay (founder of a private dispensary and nursing school) established the Association des Infirmières-Visiteuses de France. The Association offered supplementary classes and a supervised *stage* to women who already had nursing diplomas and who wished to "devote a certain amount of time per week to the care of the sick poor in their homes."[29] Lest the organization encounter resistance from private doctors, the general-secretary stressed that the *infirmières-visiteuses* "will be only auxiliaries dependent on the doctors, and will not be allowed to go to a family without the doctor's authorization in cases of illnesses that require treatment." A visiting nurse could only enter a patient's home on the recommendation of a physician. Once again, the proposed expansion of the nurse's role threatened to blur professional boundaries that were still, in the first decades of the twentieth century, coming into focus.[30]

When the war broke out six months later, the need for nurses specializing in the care of tuberculosis patients increased dramatically. The German invasion of French territory precipitated the closing or militarization of numerous sanatoria and hospitals, along with the exodus of thousands of refugees from the battle zones into the already crowded cities. In response, the Association des Infirmières-Visiteuses de France created an abbreviated version of its program in 1915 that allowed for the rapid training of large numbers of nurses specializing in tuberculosis. After only three months of classes and practical experience, graduates could serve as staff in special tubercular hospital wards, dispensaries, or temporary "sanitary stations" set up by the government near the military zone, or as visiting nurses for tubercular soldiers sent to recover in their homes.[31] In April 1916, the government passed a law mandating the creation of special dispensaries for social hygiene, dedicated particularly to educating the population about tuberculosis and its prevention. The circular that promulgated the law in 1917 called upon "specialized personnel, preferably visiting nurses" for follow-up treatments and surveillance of patients in the home, where living conditions and habits could be observed and corrected.[32]

It was the massive destruction of life during the war that brought public health and hygiene issues to the forefront of state policy. Beginning in the final years of the war and continuing into the immediate postwar era, the French government, in collaboration with the French Red Cross, the American Red Cross, and the American Rockefeller Commission, launched nationwide campaigns to combat tuberculosis. Building on the turn-of-the-century work already accomplished in Lille, Paris, and Lyons, the postwar initiatives focused on the establishment of dispensaries and centers for the instruction of proper hygiene techniques. In 1920 the government created the country's first Ministry of Hygiene, Social Assistance, and Prevention. Headed by the prominent natalist Jules-Bréton, the new ministry sponsored numerous projects to promote maternal health and *puériculture* (child-care education). The vast Maternité Baudelocque in Paris, which was devoted entirely to pre- and postnatal care, was a creation of the immediate postwar years, as was natalist Alphonse Pinard's Institut de Puériculture. In 1918 the American Red Cross sponsored an exhibit on children's hygiene and health care in Lyons that attracted over 170,000 visitors (approximately a quarter of the city's population).[33]

These postwar public health programs sought mainly to organize the instruction of proper domestic hygiene and the supervision of maternal child care—all of which were to take place primarily in the home. Thus it seemed a natural corollary that female nurses would play an essential part in implementing them. "Modern nursing is at the present time the principal need of ravaged and devastated Europe," wrote Clara D. Noyes, nursing director of the American Red Cross in 1921. France in particular "must be able to rely entirely on women to combat disease." Dr. William Welch, also of the American Red Cross, concurred, advising the international Committee of Red Cross Societies that "we can hardly think of the new activities now projected without increased nursing service."[34]

The expanded role envisioned for women in carrying out postwar public health programs centered on the care of children. The international group of doctors and health-care administrators who attended the 1919 Interallied Conference on Social Hygiene for the Reconstruction of Regions Devastated by the War (Congrès Interallié d'Hygiène Sociale pour la Reconstruction des Régions Devastées par la Guerre) identified *puériculture* and school hygiene as the two principal areas that required the services of large numbers of trained women. Adolphe Espine, vice-president of the International Committee of the Red Cross, agreed that "the woman's role is preponderant in the protection of infancy."[35] In 1919 the

American Red Cross established a foundation in France for *visiteuses* of children in their homes and a school for *puériculture,* and soon thereafter similar schools opened in Marseille, Bordeaux, and Paris. By 1921 negotiations were underway in Paris between the Institut Lannelongue and the Ministry of Public Education to set up facilities for the training of school nurses.[36]

It is indisputable that the immediate postwar period saw a dramatic flowering of opportunities for women to contribute directly to the welfare of the nation with the explicit approbation of the state. Yet the relationship between these new positions—*visiteuses d'hygiène sociale, visiteuses d'hygiène infantile, visiteuses d'écoles, visiteuses de puériculture, infirmières-visiteuses, infirmières-scolaires*—and the nursing profession remained unclear. Léonie Chaptal believed that the former constituted specialties within the field of nursing. In her 1921 report she recommended that the various *visiteuses* and school nurses be required to complete the full two-year training that she deemed necessary for all nurses, with only part of that time devoted to specialization. Not everyone agreed: Dr. Gustave Dron (senator and CSAP member) took issue with Chaptal's characterization of the new varieties of nursing as professions, noting that while the midwife, for example, was "a professional," the type of nurse/*visiteuse* that the country needed now "belongs to another social category." The *visiteuse,* in his estimation, was more a social worker than a professional nurse. The ranks of the various *visiteuses* could easily be filled by women without any nursing background, "young girls with a good up-bringing and with a general education who would be content with a modest remuneration on the condition, however, that they do not fall socially." The numerous female teachers left unemployed at the end of the war, for example, could be trained to be school nurses, an area where Dron saw particular need.[37]

The largest pool of potential candidates for the new public health and hygiene positions were the thousands of Red Cross volunteers and temporary nurses whose careers had ended with the armistice. Despite their ambiguous status as bona fide nurses, the government did not hesitate to turn to the Red Cross volunteers to fill the ranks of *visiteuses.* Indeed, CSAP president Paul Strauss regarded the Red Cross nurses as ideal candidates to become "lady patronesses, . . . *visiteuses,* or . . . instructors of infant hygiene, [or] visiting nurses." The postwar public health crisis presented "a unique opportunity to call on all those with good will, to organize them and retain them."[38] Likewise, a writer for *La Française* regarded the "numerous nurses trained in the rough school of war and currently unemployed" as potentially "indispensable auxiliaries in the struggle against the plagues" of alcoholism, infant mortality, tuberculosis, syphilis, and the like.[39]

Wealthy women and members of religious orders (all of whom worked without pay) constituted another source of female public health personnel, filling a number of the *visiteuse* and nursing positions. Nearly every city in the country depended to a degree on benevolent workers and *congréganistes* for their public health services. In Marseille, women in childbirth received visits from benevolent nurses. In Montauban, members of the local Comité de la Goutte de Lait—a charitable organization that operated infant welfare centers throughout the country—served as *visiteuses d'enfants*. Volunteers from the Red Cross UFF in Pau visited poor children in their homes, while infants in the town remained the province of the religious sisters who ran the local crèche. The city of Saint-Etienne relied on benevolent *visiteuses* supplied by the department for its maternal and infant hygiene services.[40]

The public acclaim accorded nurses during the war and the burgeoning of the public health field in the postwar years had done nothing to alter the dual characterization of nursing as paid labor and charitable work (whether of a religious or secular nature). In the half-century or so before the war, many nursing reformers had sought to draw a clear professional distinction between the untrained, unscientific members of religious nursing congregations and trained, paid, lay nurses. But the dominant presence of unpaid nurses during the war established a class and occupational split within lay nursing that undermined the efforts of those who sought to establish nursing as a respectable career comparable to teaching. The continued importance of volunteers in the social hygiene services of the postwar period, coupled with the willingness of health officials to sacrifice quality of training for quantity of nurses, continued that trend and further blurred the boundary between professional nursing and charitable duty. By creating the new roles for lay nurses the state was able to attach women's labor firmly to the government's broader social agenda, much as the recruitment of nurses during the war had linked women's work with the state's military goals. But that attachment, welcome as it was to many nurses and *visiteuses,* came at the price of growing associations between nursing and child care and between nursing and domestic hygiene, associations that transformed feminine national service into a twentieth-century version of republican motherhood.

The valorization of nursing through the expansion of state-sanctioned positions proved to be a mixed blessing for the profession. On the one hand, the importance of specifically female labor power to the national welfare was reconfirmed, and the status of paid women health-care workers rose accordingly. On the other hand, the need for the establishment of clear boundaries between professional and amateur nurses that emerged so powerfully from the war experience remained unmet. Chaptal's 1921 report centered on the importance of a state-administered nursing exam and diploma that would follow from a minimum of two full years of formal training. But the CSAP members in attendance focused almost exclusively on the need for school nurses—whose primary function would be to teach proper hygiene to children[41]—and for *visiteuses d'hygiene infantile*. For these specialties, several CSAP physicians insisted, the training period ought to be significantly shorter than that of the regular nurse; the two-year requirement would discourage too many capable young women from entering the new professions. Advocates of less instruction had powerful allies among none other than the Americans, the very standard bearers of professional nursing. The Rockefeller Institute, which funded a nationwide campaign against tuberculosis in France centered in Bordeaux, supported the reduction of training for visiting social hygiene nurses from two years to eight or nine months. Bowing to pressure from the CSAP, Chaptal quickly conceded that "for a simple specialization, six months can be allowed as a minimum."[42]

But the decree issued on June 27, 1922, establishing the official title of Licensed Nurse of the French State (*Infirmière Diplomée de l'Etat Français*) closely followed Chaptal's original recommendations. Promulgated by Paul Strauss, the former CSAP president now serving as Minister of Hygiene, the measure created *brevets de capacité* (licenses) not just for hospital nurses but also for *visiteuses d'hygiène* and nurses specializing in *puériculture,* school health inspection, mental health, and other subcategories of the profession (designated by an open-ended "etc." in the decree itself). The decree, which met with widespread approval in the general press, stipulated that aspirants to the title of Licensed Nurse complete a *stage* of at least two years at a public or private nursing school attached to a hospital whose program had been previously approved by the Minister of Hygiene. Successful candidates were also required to pass a standardized exam before a jury of representatives of the local university medical faculty and of the local practicing doctors, as well as a representative of the nursing schools and a practicing nurse.

Following Chaptal's guidelines, the measure called for the establishment of a 30-member Council for the Improvement of Nursing Schools, which would advise the Minister of Hygiene on setting the standards for approval of training programs, recommend questions for the state exam, and set the length of the *stage* required for each specialty. In no case could that training period fall below the two years required for the general nursing diploma. During the first year of the law's existence, twenty-eight schools applied for certification. Only three were approved "without reservation": Anna Hamilton's newly renamed Ecole Florence Nightingale in Bordeaux, Léonie Chaptal's Maison-Ecole d'Infirmières Privées, and the Ecole d'Infirmières de l'Hôpital Civil de Reims.[43] Perhaps not coincidentally, all three institutions had representatives on the newly created council.

In many ways the 1922 regulations constituted a clear victory for the professionalization of nursing. The two-year minimum training requirement, with its insistence on an extensive *stage* performed in a hospital, met (at least nominally) even Anna Hamilton's stringent standards.[44] Perhaps more importantly, the decree made the various new social hygiene positions into nursing specialties rather than auxiliary posts. But the law also had serious limitations. It did not mandate the state diploma as a prerequisite for employment as a nurse even in public facilities, nor did it anticipate such a requirement in the future. In other words, nursing students were free to seek out accredited schools and take the state exam but, unlike midwives, nurses did not need the state diploma to practice the profession. In addition, the powerful Council for the Improvement of Nursing Schools was dominated by physicians and health-care administrators from both private and state-run organizations. Despite Chaptal's earlier recommendation that the council include "a number of nursing school directors and qualified nurses," the group, as it was constituted in August 1922, counted among its thirty members only Anna Hamilton, the *directrice* of the Hôpital Civil de Reims, and the *directrice* of the Strasbourg nursing school, and not a single practicing nurse. The president of the original council was the eminent Paris professor of medicine, Maurice Letulle; Léonie Chaptal served as vice-president.[45] Control of the newly legitimized profession lay not with the nurses themselves but with the public health administrators (both government and private) and the physicians who dominated the council.

In the forty-four years that elapsed since the establishment of Bourneville's first municipal training programs in Paris, the nursing profession underwent substantial reform, including the laicization of a number of urban hospitals, the establishment of numerous training programs, the improvement of salaries and working conditions, and the first (albeit largely unsuccessful) attempts to define nursing as caring for patients. From an occupation that had been largely ignored by the state, nursing emerged in the closing decades of the nineteenth century as an important element in the successful operation of the hospital as a therapeutic institution. Government authorities, hospital administrators, doctors, nurses, and nursing reformers all recognized that modern medicine required nurses to be capable of more than ensuring the physical and spiritual comfort of patients. The new nurse had to be capable of understanding and implementing theories of hygiene and antisepsis, and of evaluating and treating medical illnesses and injuries within the strict parameters laid out by the medical profession.

The gradual and geographically uneven evolution of nursing from a form of religious vocation or domestic service to a health-care profession was tied inextricably to the identification of nursing as women's work. Although the field had long been associated with women's "natural" capacity for nurturing, the end of the nineteenth and beginning of the twentieth century witnessed the increasingly explicit linking of the professionalization of nursing with its simultaneous feminization. Indeed, the connection between nursing and essential femininity grew stronger as the anticlerical political climate of the period weakened the bond between nursing and religious devotion. Even the staunchest advocates of nursing as a skilled medical profession grounded their definitions of the modern nurse in contemporary notions of women's nature.

The 1922 legislation emerged from nursing leaders' desire to establish officially that nursing was a trained profession and not simply a gender attribute. Despite the prestige that nursing had acquired during the war, the bid for state licensing was intended largely as a corrective to—rather than as a confirmation of—the wartime experience. The new regulations constituted the state's response to the demand for standards in a field that seemed to bear an increasingly weak relationship to concrete training and skills, and an increasingly strong relationship to womanly duty.

Ironically, it was the advocates of professional nursing themselves who had insisted throughout the four preceding decades that the reform of nursing hinged on the feminization of the field. It was they who argued that the inherently female capacity for nurturing, gentleness, and sympathy suited women alone to carry out the duties of the professional nurse in the modern medical hospital. This invocation of innate feminine attributes conformed neatly to prevailing understandings of gendered social roles and thus served reformers well in gaining significant official and public support for the feminization of the profession. Supporters of religious and secular nursing alike could agree that nursing belonged, naturally, to women.

But reformers also insisted that nursing required both a solid basic education and extensive professional training. Here they suddenly encountered resistance, again from across the political spectrum. As long as nursing was understood to be a natural attribute of womanhood, it was deemed useful and important, yet subordinate and unthreatening. Once reformers demanded rigorous training as well as substantive authority for nurses as medical professionals, politicians, administrators, and doctors alike balked. Many objectors urged continued support for religious nursing, which remained safely within the realm of charitable work and, whatever the real expertise of the sisterhoods, never really threatened the authority of the ascendant medical profession. Those whose politics could not accommodate the presence of congregations in public hospitals, carefully limited the amount of training and the autonomy granted to lay nurses.

Of course, nursing reformers throughout Europe and the United States all faced the problem of promoting a skilled profession rooted in an essentialist identity. Nurses everywhere faced the additional challenge of establishing professional autonomy while recognizing their subordinate position in the medical hierarchy. Yet whereas by the early twentieth century English and American nurses had successfully carved out a place for themselves as medical professionals, French lay nurses faced a much more ambiguous future. Only a handful of cities had opted to follow the model provided by the Bordeaux and Paris nursing schools. Religious nurses still ran the wards of many municipal institutions and still dominated popular imagery. Lay nursing was still widely associated with charitable duty, noblesse oblige, and, for a brief period, with feminine patriotism.

In this volume I have tried to show how the particular social and political contradictions of the early Third Republic made it impossible for a secular, professional model of nursing—or any other single model—to emerge triumphant in France. The early association of professionalization with feminization and secularization meant that debates about the future of nursing would effectively be transmuted into far more fundamental disputes about the role of women in public institutions, the relationship between women and the Church, and the relationship between women's work and the family. Thus many proponents of secularized nursing worried that simultaneous professionalization and feminization would not only threaten the male medical hierarchy but displace women's central identity as mother. Many committed anticlerical politicians, doctors, and administrators found themselves favoring religious nurses who, though standing in direct contradiction to the secular foundation of the republic, constituted a known feminine form. The ideological imperatives of the Third Republic, dominated by secularization, pronatalism, and scientific progress, could find no accommodation for the professional woman who was committed first and foremost not to her family, to the Church, or even to her country, but to the public good and to her own professional advancement. Women's presence in public institutions like the hospital, unmediated by ties to Church or family (or its impoverished or military surrogates) suggested a new definition of female citizenship in which women, like men, stood as individuals in direct, unmediated relationship to the state. It was a definition that those in power were not ready to accept. Nursing reformers who had viewed the late-nineteenth-century secularizing impulse as an opportunity to create a new, respectable occupation for women failed to foresee that the feminine identity they so carefully laid out for the profession would leave them vulnerable to all the strictures associated with "the feminine." In the early decades of twentieth-century France that meant, above all, serving society as mothers.

ABBREVIATIONS USED IN THE NOTES

NOTES

INDEX

Abbreviations Used in the Notes

American Journal of Nursing	AJN
Archives de l'Assistance Publique	AAP
Archives Départementales	AD
Archives Municipales	AM
Archives Nationales	AN
British Journal of Nursing	BJN
Bulletin professionnel des infirmiers et infirmières (later renamed *Bulletin professionnel des infirmiers et des gardes-malades)*	BP
Bulletin mensuel de la Société Amicale des Surveillants et Surveillantes	BM
Conseil Supérieur de l'Assistance Publique	CSAP
La Garde-malade hospitalière	GM
La Gazette des hôpitaux	GH
Le Progrès medical	PM
La Revue philanthropique	RP

Notes

Introduction

1. *BP,* 6 (February 15, 1898): 648. (Translations from the French are my own.)
2. Until 1903, the "secondary personnel" within the hospital was generally divided into six hierarchical ranks, ranging from *surveillantes/surveillants* at the top, through *sous-surveillant(e)s, suppléant(e)s, première infirmière/infirmier, infirmière/infirmier, fille/garçon de service.* The top four ranks constituted the *personnel gradé,* and the lower two, the *personnel non-gradé.* Each rank was further divided into classes, each of which corresponded to a salary level. Henri Napias, "Rapport sur le recrutement du personnel secondaire dans les établissements hospitaliers" (1898), reprinted in CSAP, fascicule 64, p. 41.
3. *PM,* 22 (November 24, 1906): 857.
4. Jules Clarétie, "La Reposante," *Le Journal* (October 31, 1900); *PM,* 7 (January 8, 1898): 26.
5. Michelle Perrot defines a "feminine profession" as one that emerges from women's "'natural,' maternal and housewifely duties." Perrot, "Qu'est-ce qu'un métier de femme?" *Mouvement social,* 140 (July-September 1987): 3.
6. *Statistique générale de la France, Statistique annuelle des institutions d'assistance* (Paris: Imprimerie nationale, 1899, 1907, 1913). Ralph Gibson, however, estimates that the number of religious nurses peaked in 1912 at 12,887. Gibson, *A Social History of French Catholicism* (London: Routledge, 1989), p. 125. Yvonne Knibiehler, ed., *Cornettes et blouses blanches: Les Infirmières dans la société française* (Paris: Hachette, 1984), p. 9.
7. Catherine Smet argues that the nursing practiced by religious orders in the earlier part of the nineteenth century was already "professional" according to certain sociological models. Smet, "Secularization and Syndicalization: The Rise of Professional Nursing in France, 1870–1914," Ph.D. diss., University of California, San Diego, 1997.
8. "Une Ecole d'infirmières," *Le Petit Journal* (October 29, 1902).

195

9. Jacques Léonard, "Femmes, religion et médecine: Les Religieuses qui soignent en France au XIXe siècle," *Annales. Economies, Sociétés, Civilisations,* 32 (September–October 1977): 887–907.

10. Colin Jones, *The Charitable Imperative: Hospitals and Nursing in the Ancien Régime and Revolutionary France* (London: Routledge, 1989).

11. Véronique Leroux-Hugon, *Des Saintes laïques: Les Infirmières à l'aube de la Troisième République* (Paris: Sciences en situation, 1992).

12. Knibiehler, ed., *Cornettes et blouses blanches;* Marie-Françoise Collière, *Promouvoir la vie* (Paris: Interéditions, 1982); Geneviève Charles, *L'Infirmière en France d'hier à aujourd'hui* (Paris: Le Centurion, 1979).

13. Ralph Gibson, "Why Republicans and Catholics Couldn't Stand Each Other in the Nineteenth Century," in Frank Tallett and Nicholas Atkin, eds., *Religion, Society and Politics in France since 1789* (London: Hambledon Press, 1991), pp. 107–108; René Rémond, *L'Anticléricalisme en France de 1815 à nos jours* (Brussels: Editions complexe, 1985).

14. Gibson, "Why Republicans and Catholics Couldn't Stand Each Other," pp. 107–108.

15. On the national campaign to secularize education, see, for example, Sarah A. Curtis, "Lay Habits: Religious Teachers and the Secularization Crisis of 1901–1904," *French History,* 9 (1995): 478–498; Caroline Ford, "Religion and the Politics of Cultural Change in Provincial France: The Resistance in Lower Brittany," *Journal of Modern History,* 62 (March 1990): 1–30; John McManners, *Church and State in France, 1870–1914* (New York: Harper and Row, 1972), pp. 45–63; Mona Ozouf, *L'Ecole, l'église et la République, 1871–1914* (Paris: Seuil, 1982).

16. Gibson, *A Social History of French Catholicism,* pp. 104–133, esp. pp. 125–127, 133; Gibson, "Le Catholicisme et les femmes en France au XIXe siècle," *Revue d'histoire de l'église de France,* 79 (January–June 1993): 63–93; Yvonne Turin, *Femmes et religieuses au XIXe siècle: Le Féminisme en religion* (Paris: Nouvelle Cité, 1989); Claude Langlois, *Le Catholicisme au féminin: Les Congrégations françaises à supérieure générale au XIXe siècle* (Paris: Les Editions du Cerf, 1984).

17. Colin Heywood, "The Catholic Church and the Formation of the Industrial Labour Force in Nineteenth-Century France: An Interpretative Essay," *European History Quarterly,* 19 (1989): 516; Laura S. Strumingher, "'A Bas les prêtres! A Bas les couvents!': The Church and the Workers in 19th Century Lyon," *Journal of Social History,* 11 (Summer 1978): 546–553.

18. Quoted in Steven C. Hause with Anne R. Kenney, *Women's Suffrage and Social Politics in the French Third Republic* (Princeton, N.J.: Princeton University Press, 1984), p. 16.

19. On the use of confession as an instrument of clerical control especially over

women, see Theodore Zeldin, "The Conflict of Moralities: Confession, Sin and Pleasure in the Nineteenth Century," in Zeldin, ed., *Conflicts in French Society: Anticlericalism, Education, and Morals in the Nineteenth Century* (London: Allen and Unwin, 1970), pp. 13–50. See also James F. McMillan, "Religion and Gender in Modern France: Some Reflections," in Tallett and Atkin, eds., *Religion, Society and Politics in France since 1789,* pp. 55–66.

20. Jack D. Ellis, *The Physician-Legislators of France: Medicine and Politics in the Early Third Republic, 1870–1914* (Cambridge: Cambridge University Press, 1990), pp. 165, 169.

21. Gibson, *The Social History of French Catholicism,* pp. 125–126; Evelyn Bernette Ackerman, *Health Care in the Parisian Countryside, 1800–1914* (New Brunswick, N.J.: Rutgers University Press, 1990); Léonard, "Femmes, religion et médecine," pp. 887–906. Matthew Ramsey makes a related point for an earlier period in *Professional and Popular Medicine in France, 1770–1830: The Social World of Medical Practice* (Cambridge: Cambridge University Press, 1988), as does Olwen Hufton in *Women and the Limits of Citizenship in the French Revolution* (Toronto: University of Toronto Press, 1992), pp. 79–88.

22. The physician Hippolyte Jeanne argued before the Chamber of Deputies in 1903 that it was the responsibility of the state to depoliticize the issue of nursing reform by regulating nursing training, much as it regulated teacher training. His efforts had little concrete effect. *Concours médical,* May 23, 1903; Ellis, *The Physician-Legislators of France,* p. 168.

23. *GH,* March 17, 1881, p. 249; March 24, 1881, p. 273.

24. On republican criticism of women's waged labor, see Judith G. Coffin, *The Politics of Women's Work: The Paris Garment Trades, 1750–1915* (Princeton, N.J.: Princeton University Press, 1996); Mary Lynn Stewart, *Women, Work and the French State: Labour Protection and Social Patriarchy, 1879–1919* (Kingston, Ont.: McGill-Queen's University Press, 1989); Laura L. Frader, "Engendering Work and Wages: The French Labor Movement and the Family Wage," in Frader and Sonya O. Rose, eds., *Gender and Class in Modern Europe* (Ithaca, N.Y.: Cornell University Press, 1996), pp. 142–164; and the three essays on French workers in Joan Wallach Scott, *Gender and the Politics of History* (New York: Columbia University Press, 1988), pp. 93–163.

25. See William Sewell, *Work and Revolution in France: The Language of Labor from the Old Regime to 1848* (Cambridge: Cambridge University Press, 1980).

26. Hause with Kenney, *Women's Suffrage and Social Politics.*

27. For example, see the essays collected in Elinor A. Accampo, Rachel G. Fuchs, and Mary Lynn Stewart, eds., *Gender and the Politics of Social Reform in France, 1870–1914* (Baltimore, Md.: The Johns Hopkins University Press, 1995), p. 10; Judith F. Stone, "Republican Ideology, Gender, and Class: France, 1860s–1914," in Frader and Rose, eds., *Gender and Class in Modern Europe,*

pp. 238–259; Karen Offen, "Body Politics: Women, Work and the Politics of Motherhood in France, 1920–1950," in Gisela Bock and Pat Thane, eds., *Maternity and Gender Policies: Women and the Rise of the European Welfare States, 1880s–1950s* (London: Routledge, 1991); "Population and the State in the Third Republic," a special issue of *French Historical Studies,* 19 (Spring 1996). Critical to understanding the gendered roots of welfare policy is Susan Pedersen, *Family, Dependence, and the Origins of the Welfare State: Britain and France, 1914–1945* (Cambridge: Cambridge University Press, 1993).

28. The law of August 7, 1851, made official the distinction between hospices and hospitals that had functioned in practice in most large cities throughout the nineteenth century. The law mandated that in the interest of the more effective use of modern therapeutic medicine, hospitals be reserved for the sick, and hospices for the old, infirm, and incurable. Many smaller institutions ignored the regulation, prompting the Minister of the Interior to issue a circular in 1899 stressing the need to separate the two kinds of patients either in different institutions or in separate services in a single hospital-hospice. Jean Imbert, *Histoire des hôpitaux en France* (Toulouse: Editions Privat, 1982), pp. 337–338.

29. Letter from Hôtel-Dieu patient Elisa Réol, March 16, 1906, AD, Rhône 1X2.

30. It was not until the 1890s, for example, that the Hospice des Enfants Assistés (for foundlings) began to separate children with contagious diseases from healthy children. Rachel Ginnis Fuchs, *Abandoned Children: Foundlings and Child Welfare in Nineteenth Century France* (Albany, N.Y.: State University of New York Press, 1984), p. 149.

31. Jules Clarétie, *La Vie à Paris,* quoted in S. Borsa and C. R. Michel, *La Vie quotidienne des hôpitaux en France au XIXe siècle* (Paris: Hachette, 1985), p. 49.

32. Ibid.

33. Ackerman, *Health Care in the Parisian Countryside;* Robert A. Nye, *Crime, Madness, and Politics in Modern France: The Medical Concept of National Decline* (Princeton, N.J.: Princeton University Press, 1984); Jacques Donzelot, *The Policing of Families* (New York: Pantheon, 1979).

34. Ackerman, *Health Care in the Parisian Countryside,* p. 123.

35. Borsa and Michel, *La Vie quotidienne,* pp. 47–74; Marcel Candille, "Les Soins en France au XIXe siècle," *Bulletin de la société française d'histoire des hôpitaux,* 28 (1974): 33–77; Imbert, *Histoire des hôpitaux en France,* pp. 337–347.

36. Letter from Assistance Publique director Henri Monod to Minister of the Interior Floquet, 1889, CSAP, fascicule 64.

37. The CSAP was composed of physicians, politicians, and administrators. See Ellis, *The Physician-Legislators of France,* pp. 224, 282, n78.

38. Emile Combes, *Circulaire du 28 octobre 1902,* CSAP fascicule 69, p. 2.

39. Henri Monod, *Circulaire du 17 juillet 1899,* CSAP fascicule 69, p. 11.

40. Hermann Sabran, quoted in *Circulaire du 17 juillet 1899,* CSAP, fascicule 64, p. 10.

41. Quoted in Borsa and Michel, *La Vie quotidienne,* p. 181.

42. Ministère de l'Intérieur et des Cultes, Direction de l'Assistance et de l'Hygiène Publique, *Circulaire du 28 octobre 1902,* CSAP fascicule 69, p. 1.

43. On the range of practitioners who provided health services to the French population in the nineteenth and early twentieth centuries and the medical profession's efforts to control the field, see Martha Hildreth, *Doctors, Bureaucrats, and Public Health in France, 1888–1902* (New York: Garland, 1987); Jacques Léonard, *La France médicale au XIXe siècle* (Paris: Gallimard-Julliard "Archives," 1978), and *La Médecine entre les pouvoirs et les savoirs: Histoire intellectuelle et politique de la médecine française au XIXe siècle* (Paris: Aubier, 1981); and Ramsey, *Professional and Popular Medicine in France.*

44. Although the demographics of all religious congregations tended toward democratization during the nineteenth century, the nursing congregations drew especially heavily from the rural, peasant population. Gibson, *Social History of French Catholicism,* p. 117; Langlois, *Le Catholicisme au féminin,* pp. 611–625.

1. Hospital Nursing in Paris

1. *L'Illustration,* January 18, 1908.

2. Ceremony at Salpêtrière, 1884, *Procès-verbaux des distributions de prix* (hereafter *Procès-verbaux),* AAP, vol. 2, p. 74; Ceremony at Salpêtrière, 1889, *Procès-verbaux,* vol. 2, p. 107.

3. The historiography of educational reform during this period is vast. See, for example, Linda L. Clark, *Schooling the Daughters of Marianne: Textbooks and the Socialization of Girls in Modern French Primary Schools* (Albany, N.Y.: State University of New York Press, 1984); Caroline Ford, "Religion and the Politics of Cultural Change in Provincial France: The Resistance of 1902 in Lower Brittany," *The Journal of Modern History,* 62 (March 1990): 1–33; Françoise Mayeur, *L'Education des filles en France au XIXe siècle* (Paris: Hachette, 1979); Antoine Prost, *Histoire de l'enseignement en France, 1800–1967* (Paris: A. Colin, 1968). For a broader discussion of Church-state relations, see Gérard Cholvy and Yves-Marie Hilaire, *Histoire religieuse de la France contemporaine,* vol. 2, *1880–1930* (Toulouse: Editions Privat, 1986), pp. 21–33, 57–105; Maurice Larkin, *Church and State after the Dreyfus Affair: The Separation Issue in France* (New York: Barnes and Noble, 1974); John McManners, *Church and State in France, 1870–1914* (New York: Harper and

Row, 1972), esp. pp. 45–63; René Rémond, *L'Anticléricalisme en France de 1815 à nos jours* (Paris: Editions Complexe, 1976).

4. See Michel Poisson, "Désiré Magloire Bourneville et les écoles municipales parisiennes d'infirmiers et d'infirmières, 1870–1900," M.A. thesis, Université de Paris VIII, Saint-Denis, 1990.

5. Charles Quentin, "Rapport du Directeur de l'Administration Générale de l'Assistance Publique au Conseil de Surveillance," December 30, 1880, AAP, folder 729²; see also a letter from Senator and physician Paul Cornil, quoted in *L'Eclair,* May 2, 1890.

6. Ralph Gibson, *A Social History of French Catholicism, 1789–1914* (London: Routledge, 1989), pp. 131–132.

7. The issue of "liberté de la conscience" was less central in Paris than, for example, in Lyons, where the sisters' purported intolerance and coercive treatment of the patients formed the basis of much of the municipal council's case against the *soeurs hospitalières.* (See Chapter 2.)

8. *Procès-verbaux du Conseil Municipal de Paris,* January 28, 1885.

9. Dr. Lezoux, quoted in Charles Quentin, "Rapport du Directeur de l'Administration Générale," December 30, 1880.

10. Excerpted from letter from Director of Les Tournelles, December 18, 1880, in "Rapport du Directeur de l'Administration Générale," December 30, 1880.

11. *Procès-verbaux du Conseil Municipal de Paris,* July 31, 1880; Ceremony at Salpêtrière, 1880, *Procès-verbaux,* vol. 1, p. 49.

12. *GH,* 22 (February 22, 1881): 169.

13. Ceremony at Salpêtrière, 1884, *Procès-verbaux,* vol. 2, p. 79.

14. *GH,* 32 (March 17, 1881): 249.

15. Ibid., and *GH,* 35 (March 24, 1881): 273.

16. *L'Eclair,* May 2, 1890.

17. Gibson, *A Social History of French Catholicism,* p. 126. See also Poisson, "Désiré Magloire Bourneville et les écoles municipales," p. 123.

18. Yvonne Knibiehler, ed., *Cornettes et blouses blanches: Les Infirmières dans la société française, 1880–1980* (Paris: Hachette, 1984), p. 16.

19. Letter from Desprès to Bourneville, March 7, 1881, in Armand Desprès, *Les Soeurs hospitalières: Lettres et discours sur la laicisation des hôpitaux* (Paris: Ancienne Maison Michel Levy Frères, 1886), p. 14. On the conflict between Desprès and Bourneville, see Pierre Guillaume, *Médecins, Eglise et foi, XIXe–XXe siècles* (Paris: Editions Aubier, 1990), pp. 82–87; Jacques Léonard, *La Médecine entre les pouvoirs et les savoirs* (Paris: Editions Aubier, 1981), pp. 288–289; Poisson, "Désiré Magloire Bourneville et les écoles municipales," pp. 103–128.

20. See, for example, *PM,* 12 (December 27, 1890): 521–525; and *PM,* 13 (January 3, 1891): 17–20.

21. Desprès, Letter to the Prefect of the Seine, February 19, 1881, reprinted in *GH*, 22 (February 22, 1881): 169; *La Leçon de Charcot: Voyage dans une toile,* Exhibition Catalogue, Musée de l'Assistance Publique de Paris, September 17-December 31, 1986, p. 113.

22. Letter from Desprès to President of Municipal Council, April 7, 1884, in Desprès, *Les Soeurs hospitalières,* p. 55; Desprès, Letter to the Prefect of the Seine, February 19, 1881.

23. "Discours sur la laicisation de l'Hospice des Enfants Assistés," November 6, 1885, in Desprès, *Les Soeurs hospitalières,* p. 160.

24. It is ironic that Desprès would stress this point, since he was one of the few Parisian surgeons to reject Lister's work on antiseptic surgical techniques. Until his death, he refused to recognize the value of sterilizing instruments or disinfecting bandages or his own hands.

25. "Discours prononcé à la réunion publique de la salle Favié à Belleville," January 30, 1886, in Desprès, *Les Soeurs hospitalières,* pp. 223–224.

26. "Chambre de Députés, séance du 20 December 1890," *PM*, 12 (December 27, 1890): 523–524; Letter to Hérold, Prefect of the Seine, February 19, 1881, in Desprès, *Les Soeurs hospitalières,* pp. 4–7.

27. Dr. Potain, "La Laicisation des hôpitaux, Necker Hospital," *L'Univers*, March 1, 1881, in AAP, Fosseyeux 646, vol. 36, p. 26. See also *La Leçon de Charcot, Voyage dans une toile,* pp. 113–114.

28. Ceremony at Salpêtrière, 1900, *Procès-verbaux,* vol. 3, p. 65. Unfortunately, available statistics do not specify the actual functions of these employees. No doubt a greater percentage of the men than of the women were employed in non-caregiving positions. At the lower levels, this might mean jobs that involved transporting patients or equipment, or strenuous cleaning. In the higher ranks of *surveillants* or *suppléants,* men might be found in greater numbers in some of the general services, in administration, or as assistants in surgical operations.

29. CSAP, *Procès-verbal de la première session d'ordinaire de 1899,* May 17, 1899, in CSAP, fascicule 64, pp. 23–24.

30. Ceremony at Salpêtrière, 1882, *Procès-verbaux,* vol. 1, p. 74.

31. Henri Napias, "Rapport sur le recrutement du personnel secondaire," CSAP, fascicule 64, (1898) p. 24; Ceremony at la Pitié, 1895, *Procès-verbaux,* vol. 3, p. 101.

32. Dr. Faivre, "Rapport présenté au nom de la IIe section: Programme de l'enseignement professionnel pour les écoles d'infirmiers et d'infirmières," CSAP, fascicule 69 (1899), p. 12.

33. Julien Noir, Ceremony at Bicêtre, 1905, *Procès-verbaux,* vol. 4, p. 13.

34. AAP, Fosseyeux 728, "Personnel congréganiste," dossier 3; *L'Illustration,* January 18, 1908; Ceremony at Salpetrière, 1893, *Procès-verbaux,* vol. 3, p. 132;

Conseil d'Etat Section du Contentieux, *Memoires pour les Soeurs de l'Hôpital Saint-Louis contre l'Administration de l'Assistance Publique* (Versailles, 1892).

35. "Proposition à l'admission des religieuses dans les services hôpitaux de la Ville de Paris et du Département de la Seine," March 12, 1913, Municipal Council Publication 11; "On propose de remplacer les infirmières par des religieuses," *Bulletin mensuel de l'Association Amicale du Personnel Gradé*, 82 (October 1913): 14–16; *La Bataille syndicale*, December 3, 1913 and December 9, 1913, in AN F⁷ 13814. For a discussion of the nursing unions' response to the threat of *reintégration*, see Chapter 4.

36. See, for example, Désiré Magloire Bourneville, "La Laicisation des hôpitaux de Paris," *Conseil international des nurses (gardes-malades), Conférence du Nursing, La troisième séance de tous congrès internationaux des nurses, Paris, 18–22 June 1907*, pp. 13–15, in Papers of the American Nurses' Association, Proceedings of the Conferences of the International Council of Nursing. The debate over the economic advantages and disadvantages of religious and lay nurses was interminable, tedious, and ultimately inconclusive, with each side manipulating budgetary figures to produce the desired results. Recent historical works that discuss the limitations of religious sisters' medical capacity include Jan Goldstein, *Console and Classify: The French Psychiatric Profession in the Nineteenth Century* (Chicago: University of Chicago Press, 1986), pp. 197–230, esp. p. 217 and Léonard, "Femmes, religion, et médecine," esp. pp. 894–895.

37. Charles Quentin, "Note sur les écoles professionnelles d'infirmiers et infirmières, 2 August 1880," in AAP, Fosseyeux 613, carton B.

38. Ceremony at Bicêtre, 1880, *Procès-verbaux*, vol. 1, p. 78.

39. Péan de Saint-Gilles, "Rapport de la Commission instituée pour examiner la question de savoir s'il y a lieu de remplacer par des laïques les soeurs qui devaient être appelées à desservir l'hôpital Ménilmontant," undated, quoted in Bourneville, Conseil Municipal de Paris, Rapport 56, [August 6] 1878, pp. 2–3, in AAP, Fosseyeux 613, box B.

40. The terms *infirmière* and *infirmier*, today translated as "nurse," were much less specific during the period under consideration here, and especially before the 1903 reforms. The title had no particular set of duties attached to it. An *infirmière* might treat patients in a ward, or she might serve food in the kitchen or sort laundry in the *buandérie*.

41. Ceremony at Bicêtre, 1880, *Procès-verbaux*, vol. 1, p. 78. A separate session was soon set up for those "already possessing a certain degree of instruction." Bourneville, Rapport 57, Conseil Municipal de Paris, [August 6] 1878, pp. 3–4.

42. Letter from Director of Bicêtre to Director of Assistance Publique, May 18, 1878, AAP, Fosseyeux 613, box B; Bourneville, "La Laicisation des hôpitaux de Paris," *Conseil international des nurses* (1907), p. 21; Ceremony at

Salpêtrière, 1888, *Procès-verbaux*, vol. 2, p. 64; Ceremony at Salpêtrière, 1889, *Procès-verbaux*, vol. 2, p. 89.

43. Charles Quentin, "Organisation des écoles d'infirmiers et d'infirmières, Rapport à Monsieur le Senateur Préfet de la Seine," 1880, AAP, Fosseyeux 613, box B; Ceremony at Salpêtrière, 1880, *Procès-verbaux*, vol. 1, p. 37; Bourneville, Conseil Municipal de Paris, Rapport 57, pp. 3–5.

44. In 1877 Bourneville joined a delegation from the Paris Municipal Council on a trip to England, which included visits to several hospitals. A few months after returning, he submitted his proposal for municipal nursing schools. "Le Doctor Bourneville," *RP*, 25 (June 15, 1909): 176; "La Laicisation des hôpitaux de Paris," *Conseil international des nurses*, (1907), p. 13.

45. Arrêté de l'Assistance Publique, November 5, 1880, in AAP, Fosseyeux 613, box B.

46. Regulations of municipal nursing schools at Bicêtre, Salpêtrière, and La Pitié, October 11, 1881; "Note sur l'école des infirmières de la Salpêtrière" (undated); "Notes sur les Ecoles d'infirmières et infirmiers à Bicêtre et Salpêtrière," January 16, 1881, all in AAP, Fosseyeux 613, box B. By 1898, primary school classes were offered in eight institutions, and professional classes in four. Napias, "Recrutement du personnel secondaire," p. 44.

47. Ceremony at La Pitié, 1881, *Procès-verbaux*, vol. 1, pp. 95–96; Ceremony at La Pitié, 1882, *Procès-verbaux*, vol. 1, pp. 102–103.

48. Ceremony at Salpêtrière, 1883, *Procès-verbaux*, vol. 1, p. 69. Ceremony at Bicêtre, 1890, *Procès-verbaux*, vol. 2, p. 37.

49. Ceremony at Salpêtrière, 1884, *Procès-verbaux*, vol. 2, p. 82; Ceremony at La Pitié, 1884, *Procès-verbaux*, p. 121; Ceremony at Lariboisière, 1896, *Procès-verbaux*, vol. 4, p. 77.

50. Ceremonies at Bicêtre, Salpêtrière, and La Pitié, 1887, 1892, *Procès-verbaux*, vols. 2, 3.

51. The statistic for educational degrees assumes that each employee held only one certificate or diploma. If, in fact, some held several degrees, then the percentage could fall as low as one-fifth. Ceremony at Salpêtrière, 1900, reprinted in *PM*, 13 (February 23, 1901): 135–136.

52. Bourneville commentary on 1902 Circular from Ministry of the Interior, AAP, Fosseyeux 646, vol. 25; *BP*, 3 (August 15, 1895): 282.

53. "A Méditer," *BP*, 3 (November 15, 1895).

54. Ceremony at Salpêtrière, 1894, *Procès-verbaux*, vol. 3, p. 102. Ceremony at Lariboisière, 1905, AAP, Fosseyeux 646, vol. 34, p. 11; Ceremony at Salpêtrière, 1893, *Procès-verbaux*, vol. 3, p. 105.

55. *BP*, 13 (October 15, 1905): 112.

56. Excerpts from "Délibérations du Conseil Municipal," June 29, 1900, *PM*, 12 (July 7, 1900): 5.

57. Circular from Assistance Publique to all hospital directors, September 28, 1905, AAP, Fosseyeux 613, box A.

58. Dr. Faivre, "Rapport présenté au nom de la IIe section," pp. 8–9; *Procès-verbal de la première session ordinaire de 1899,* CSAP, fascicule 69, pp. 7–40.

59. The phrase "vaillantes filles du peuple" comes from a 1905 speech by Dr. Julien Noir, one of Bourneville's staunchest defenders. Noir argued passionately for recruiting nurses from among the lower classes, in direct disagreement with Anna Hamilton's proposals (see Chapter 3). Ceremony at Bicêtre, 1905, AAP, Fosseyeux 646, vol. 34, p. 13.

60. The Nationalists won 45 out of 80 seats, ousting the Socialist-Radicals (Bourneville's political allies) from power. Jean-Marie Mayeur and Madeleine Rebérieux, *The Third Republic from Its Origins to the Great War, 1871–1914* (Cambridge: Cambridge University Press, 1987), p. 206.

61. *Procès-verbaux du Conseil Municipal de Paris,* June 29, 1900, reprinted in *PM,* 12 (July 7, 1900): 6.

62. Ibid. pp. 5–12; *PM,* 13 (January 12, 1901): 20–22.

63. *L'Aurore,* January 2, 1901; *Le Petit Sou,* November 29, 1900; *PM,* 13 (January 12, 1901): 22; Letter from Prefect of the Seine to Director of Assistance Publique, February 26, 1901, AAP, Fosseyeux 613, box B.

64. Napias, "Rapport sur le recrutement du personnel secondaire," p. 11. Annual salaries for the top five ranks of employees ranged from about 400 francs for *infirmières* and *infirmiers* to about 900 francs for *surveillantes* and *surveillants,* in addition to room and board. Victor Trichet, "La Réforme du personnel hospitalier à l'Assistance Publique de Paris," *RP,* 12 (February 10, 1903): 463.

65. Trichet, "La Réforme du personnel hospitalier," p. 453.

66. *BP,* 10 (July 15, 1902): 1281.

67. Ceremony at Salpêtrière, 1900; *PM,* 13 (February 23, 1901): 136.

68. Trichet, "La Réforme du personnel hospitalier," pp. 453–454.

69. Ceremony at Lariboisière, 1896, reprinted in *PM,* 4 (October 10, 1896): 241.

70. *BP,* 10 (July 15, 1902): 1281.

71. Commission du Conseil de Surveillance chargée d'étudier le projet de réorganisation du personnel hospitalier, séance du 26 June 1902, in Administration Générale de l'Assistance Publique à Paris, *Réorganisation du personnel hospitalier* (Montévrain: Imprimérie de l'Ecole d'Alembert, 1904), p. 221; *RP,* 1 (August 10, 1897).

72. *Réorganisation du personnel hospitalier,* p. 221.

73. Henri Napias, Ceremony at Salpêtrière, 1899, *Procès-verbaux,* vol. 4, p. 26.

74. Commission . . . de réorganisation du personnel hospitalier, *Procès-verbaux des séances,* February 19, 1902–April 21, 1902, in *Réorganisation du personnel hospitalier,* p. 70.

75. Commission du Conseil de Surveillance, April 27, 1902, *Réorganisation du personnel hospitalier,* pp. 153–154.

76. Commission du Conseil de Surveillance, February 25, 1902, *Réorganisation du personnel hospitalier*, p. 80.

77. Jo Burr Margadant, *Madame le Professeur: Women Educators in the Third Republic* (Princeton: Princeton University Press, 1990), pp. 40, 62–82.

78. Commission du Conseil de Surveillance, February 25, 1902, *Réorganisation du personnel hospitalier*, p. 81.

79. The director of Assistance Publique for the city pointed to the existing dormitories as proof that institutional residence in and of itself did not guarantee better discipline or stricter behavioral codes. *BP*, 10 (July 15, 1902): 1281.

80. For the perspectives of the various nurses' unions and associations on this issue, see Chapter 4.

81. "Inauguration de l'Ecole des Infirmières de l'Assistance Publique," *BM*, 40 (December 1908): 30.

82. "Les Nouveaux Hôpitaux de Paris: L'Ecole d'infirmières," draft of brochure, in AM, Lyons, Q³, uncatalogued.

83. Hamilton, *Considérations sur les infirmières des hôpitaux*, pp. 125–135; Paul-Louis Lande, "Chronique: Mise au point," *GM*, 28 (January 1909): 11; "L'Ecole de la Salpêtrière," *GM*, 29 (February 1909): 27–34.

84. "L'Ecole de la Salpêtrière," pp. 25–26.

85. In 1905 Hamilton voiced her objections to the creation of a National Council of French Nurses, which would be represented at the International Council of Nurses, on the grounds that such a group would undoubtedly only reflect the ideas of "the parisian (sic) 'mondaine' or the 'official' assistance publique." Letters from Hamilton to Lavinia Dock, November 28, 1905 and December 29, 1907, in M. Adelaide Nutting Papers, Teachers College, Columbia University, microfiche no. 2442.

86. *Ecole des Infirmières de l'Assistance Publique de Paris* (1909, no publication information), p. 9.

87. "L'Ecole des Infirmières de l'Assistance Publique," *BP*, 16 (June 15, 1908): 62. See also "Ecole des Infirmières de l'Assistance Publique," *RP*, 23 (October 15, 1908): 755.

88. *Ecole des infirmières de l'Assistance Publique de Paris*, p. 10.

89. *BP*, 16 (June 15, 1908): 64; "Ecole des Infirmières de l'Assistance Publique," p. 755. See also André Mesureur, "L'Ecole des Infirmières de l'Assistance Publique," *L'Illustration* (September 5, 1908): 159.

90. *Ecole des Infirmières de l'Assistance Publique*, p. 9.

91. *BM*, 40 (December 1908): 25.

92. Quoted in "L'Assistance Publique de Paris: La Formation du personnel," *Les Nouvelles*, August 16, 1909, in AAP, Fosseyeux 613, box B.

93. *BM*, 40 (December 1908): 29–31. See also *AJN*, 9 (February 1909): 356.

94. *BP*, 11 (September 15, 1903): 1445.

95. The Augustine Sisters of the Hôtel-Dieu were not the first religious nurses to

attend the programs. In 1902 eight sisters from the Augustines of the Sacred-Heart of Mary (not affiliated with the Augustines of the Hôtel-Dieu) completed the program and received diplomas. These women ran a private hospital in Paris. *Le Petit Journal,* December 1, 1903.

96. Ceremony at Bicêtre, 1905, AAP, Fosseyeux 646, vol. 34, p. 12.

97. "L'Ecole des Infirmières," *RP,* 30 (April 15, 1912): 647–648.

98. *BP,* 14 (August 15, 1906): 92.

99. *BP,* 14 (June 15, 1906): 70; *GM* (February 1909): 31.

100. *Fédération des Services de Santé de France et des Colonies, IIe Congrès corporatif, 28–30 September-1 October 1908* (Bourges: Imprimerie ouvrière du centre ouvriers, syndiqués, et fédérés, 1908), pp. 30–31.

101. Abadie used the phrase "diplôme féminin ou des nurses," deliberately employing the English word "nurse" to suggest the Anglo-American model of a middle-class ladies' profession. *Fédération des Services de Santé de France et des Colonies, IIe Congrès corporatif,* pp. 30–31. For a discussion of Abadie and the Fédération, see Chapter 4.

102. M. Honoré, memo dated November 15, 1913, Minutes of the CSAP, December 4, 1913, p. 159.

103. *L'Action,* October 6, 1908, in AN F⁷13813; *La Réforme du personnel hospitalier (1903–1910): Ecole des Infirmières de l'Assistance Publique de Paris* (1909, no publication information), f.n. 16.

104. *Ecole des Infirmières de l'Assistance Publique de Paris* (Montevrain: Imprimérie de l'Ecole d'Alembert, 1912), pp. 34–35.

105. *Procès-verbaux du Conseil de Surveillance de l'Assistance Publique de Paris,* March 8, 1923, p. 425.

106. *Les Nouvelles,* August 16, 1909, in AAP, Fosseyeux 613, box B.

107. "Inauguration de l'Ecole des Infirmières de l'Assistance Publique à l'Hospice de la Salpêtrière," *BM,* 40 (December 1908): 33. See also *Le Journal des débats* (November 5, 1908).

2. The Nursing Sisters of Lyons

1. In 1899 the Ministry of Commerce, Industry, and Postal and Telegraph Services listed 12,108 religious hospital workers, 1,132 of whom worked in the department of the Rhône. The statistics, compiled from a survey sent out to the prefects, revealed an increase in religious nurses from the approximately 10,000 under the Second Empire. *Statistique générale de la France, Statistique annuelle des institutions d'assistance, 1899* (Paris: Imprimerie nationale, 1902). See also Evelyne Diebolt, *La Maison de Santé Protestante de Bordeaux (1863–1934)* (Toulouse: Erès, 1990), pp. 68–69; André Latreille, "La Vie politique et le mouvement des idées de 1815 à 1905," in Latreille, ed., *Histoire*

de Lyon et du Lyonnais (Toulouse: Privat, 1975), p. 342; Ralph Gibson, *A Social History of French Catholicism, 1789–1914* (London: Routledge, 1989), p. 105; Claude Langlois, *Le Catholicisme au féminin: Les Congrégations françaises à supérieure générale au XIXe siècle* (Paris: Les Editions du Cerf, 1984), p. 321.

2. Anna Emilie Hamilton, "Considérations sur les infirmières des hôpitaux," MD thesis, Medical School of Montpellier, 1900, p. 119. The thesis was later published and ensuing references will be to the published work.

3. Banned by decree on August 18, 1792, the Sisters of Charity remained for the most part in hospital service, though not as congregation members. On 1re nivôse IX (January 22, 1801) religious nurses were officially allowed to return to the hospitals, and the Sisters of Charity were again legally recognized by Charles X in 1825. Langlois, *Le Catholicisme au féminin*, p. 523. For the history of the Sisters of Charity through the first half of the nineteenth century, see Colin Jones, "The Filles de la Charité in Hospitals," in *Vincent de Paul: Actes du colloque international d'études vincentiennes*, Paris, September 25–26, 1981 (Rome: C.L.V. Edizioni Vincenziane, 1983), pp. 239–288, and his *The Charitable Imperative: Hospitals and Nursing in the Ancien Régime and Revolutionary France* (London: Routledge, 1989). See also Jacques Léonard, "Femmes, religion et médecine: Les Religieuses qui soignent en France au XIXe siècle," *Annales, Société, Economie, Civilisation*, 32 (September-October 1977): 887–907; *Les Filles de la Charité de Saint Vincent de Paul* (Paris: Letouzey et Ané, 1923).

4. Speech delivered at the Hospice de l'Antiquaille, April 26, 1891, M. E. Caillemer, *Discours prononcés à l'occasion des croisures des soeurs hospitalières* (Lyons, 1913), p. 8 (hereafter *Discours*).

5. "Une Ecole d'infirmières," *Le Petit Journal*, October 29, 1902, in Archives des Hospices Civils de Lyon (hereafter cited as HCL Archives), file: "Ecole d'Infirmières."

6. "L'Organisation hospitalière lyonnaise," *RP*, 1 (December 10, 1897): 265.

7. Deliberations of General Administrative Council of the Hospices Civils de Lyon (hereafter cited as GAC HCL), November 18, 1885.

8. Extrait du Régistre des Délibérations, GAC HCL, January 28, 1880.

9. Deliberations of GAC HCL, *croisure* at Hôtel-Dieu, July 25, 1883.

10. Extrait du Régistre des Délibérations, GAC HCL, January 28, 1880.

11. "L'Organisation hospitalière lyonnaise," *RP*, 1 (December 10, 1897): 264.

12. Auguste Croze, *Les Soeurs hospitalières des Hospices Civils de Lyon* (Lyon: Impressions de M. Augin, 1933), p. 22. See also Natalie Zemon Davis, "Scandale à l'Hôtel-Dieu de Lyon (1537–1543)," in *La France d'Ancien Régime: Etudes réunies en l'honneur de Pierre Goubert* (Toulouse: Privat, 1984), vol. 1, pp. 175–187.

13. In 1880 there were 127 brothers in all HCL institutions, 41 in medical services, and 86 serving in other capacities. By 1910 only 27 *hospitaliers* remained, all in non-sickcare positions. The last two *frères hospitaliers* entered the Hôtel-Dieu in 1898. *Comptes morales administratifs des Hospices Civils de Lyon,* 1880, 1890, 1900, 1910, in HCL Archives; *Histoire du Grand Hôtel-Dieu de Lyon des origines à l'année 1900* (Lyons: Audin, 1924), p. 217.

14. Extrait du Registre des Délibérations, GAC HCL, January 28, 1880, p. 2.

15. Davis, "Scandale à l'Hôtel-Dieu de Lyon," p. 178.

16. William Monter notes that during the years immediately following the Council of Trent, "many convents continued to serve as dumping-grounds for surplus daughters of Catholic aristocrats." Monter, "Protestant Wives, Catholic Saints, and the Devil's Handmaid: Women in the Age of Reformations," in Renate Bridenthal, Claudia Koonz, Susan Stuard, eds., *Becoming Visible: Women in European History,* 2nd ed. (Boston: Houghton Mifflin, 1987), p. 209. On the more democratic social origins of members of congregations in the nineteenth century, see Gibson, *A Social History of French Catholicism,* pp. 116–117; Langlois, *Le Catholicisme au féminin,* pp. 611–625; Hazel Mills, "Negotiating the Divide: Women, Philanthropy and the 'Public Sphere' in Nineteenth-Century France," in Frank Tallett and Nicholas Atkin, eds., *Religion, Society and Politics in France since 1789* (London: Hambledon Press, 1991), p. 45.

17. Jean-Antoine-Claude Chaptal, *Mes souvenirs sur Napoléon* (Paris: E. Plon, Nourrit, 1893), p. 72, quoted in M. E. Caillemer, *Les Hospices Civils de Lyon, leur administration* (Lyons: 1910), p. 102.

18. M. Trolliet, *Compte-rendu des obsérvations faites à l'Hôtel-Dieu de Lyon, 1822–1824* (Lyons: Durand, 1825), quoted in Olivier Faure, *Genèse de l'hôpital moderne: Les Hospices Civils de Lyon de 1802 à 1845* (Lyons: Presses universitaires de Lyon, 1982), p. 111.

19. Faure, *Genèse de l'hôpital moderne,* pp. 155–156.

20. Caillemer, *Les Hospices Civils de Lyon, leur administration,* pp. 142–143; Caillemer, *Discours,* pp. 33–34. The Sisters of Charity continued to staff Lyons' military hospital throughout the period under consideration, but the institution did not belong to the HCL.

21. Faure, *La Genèse de l'hôpital moderne,* pp. 154–155. For a complete account of the documents relating to the incident, see Marcel Colly, "L'Affaire Gabriel à l'Hôtel-Dieu, 1830–1834," *Albums du crocodile* (March-April, 1959). A similar though less famous incident occurred in 1830, immediately after the July Revolution. Caillemer, *Discours,* p. 50.

22. Deliberations of GAC HCL, May 24, 1904.

23. Caillemer, *croisure* of Croix-Rousse Hospital, April 16, 1893, *Discours,* p. 12.

24. Deliberations of GAC HCL, October 30, 1889.

25. Deliberations of GAC HCL, November 10, 1920. The need for a pension plan for nurses would become a central demand of the nurses' unions.

26. On November 13, 1915, the government declared that all Austro-German *religieuses* had to leave French soil. Soeur Merck became a naturalized citizen after the war and rejoined the Hôtel-Dieu staff. Deliberations of GAC HCL, November 7, 1915; February 23, 1916; October 4, 1916; February 6, 1918; April 16, 1919; May 5, 1920; December 29, 1920. See also Brizon, *Causérie sur les soeurs hospitalières des Hospices Civils de Lyon* (Lyons, 1940), p. 30.

27. Deliberations of GAC HCL, March 4, 1908.

28. Deliberations of GAC HCL, March 25, 1903. By the beginning of the next decade, the GAC began to see the home visits as occasions for recruiting novices to shore up the dwindling ranks of young nurses. Caillemer, *croisures* at Asile Ste.-Eugénie, July 2, 1911, and at Hôtel-Dieu, January 24, 1912, in *Discours,* pp. 55–57.

29. Personnel folders of Charité Hospital, HCL Archives. These records, which exist only for the Charité and the Hôtel-Dieu, are statistically unreliable. Most of the folders offer only the name and date of entry and departure. Some give the reason for departure (illness, death, or voluntary) and place of birth, and a few give the father's occupation.

30. Between 1899 and 1905, of 137 *hospitalières* who received a cross for 12–15 years of service, 75 percent were age 20 or older when they entered service.

31. AM, Lyons, box Q3, uncatalogued.

32. A second-degree midwife diploma entitled the holder to practice only in the province where the degree was issued, whereas the more rigorous training leading to the first degree diploma allowed the recipient to practice anywhere in France.

33. For an evocative discussion of the peculiar hazards of being a poor woman in a nineteenth-century French city, see Rachel G. Fuchs, *Poor and Pregnant in Paris: Strategies for Survival in the Nineteenth Century* (New Brunswick, N.J.: Rutgers University Press, 1992).

34. In Lyons, the Progréssistes were popularly referred to as the Parti Aynard.

35. Guy Laperrière, *La "Séparation" à Lyon (1904–1908): Etude d'opinion publique* (Grenoble: Presses universitaires, 1973), p. 77.

36. David Lathoud, *Une Ame de miséricorde, Soeur Jeanne Aynard, hospitalière de l'Hôtel-Dieu de Lyon* (Lyons: Librairie Catholique Emmanuel Vitte, 1937).

37. Ibid., pp. 84–85.

38. Ibid., p. 159.

39. Ibid., p. 148.

40. Ibid., p. 172.

41. On the role of the congregations as arenas for feminine association and as organizations that provided rare opportunities for female social action, see

Odile Arnold, *Le Corps et l'âme: La Vie des religieuses au XIXe siècle* (Paris: Editions du Seuil, 1984), pp. 168–169; Gibson, *A Social History of French Catholicism*, pp. 117–119; Yvonne Turin, *Femmes et religieuses au XIXe siècle: Le Féminisme en religion* (Paris: Nouvelle Cité, 1989); see also Mills, "Negotiating the Divide," pp. 43–46.

42. Latreille, "La Vie politique et le mouvement des idées," pp. 340–347.
43. HCL archives, personnel files of la Charité.
44. *Le Progrès,* September 14, 1880.
45. AD, Rhône, 1X2.
46. *Lyon Républicain,* April 13, 1881.
47. AD, Rhône, 1Xp 228.
48. The administration even asked the Prefect to send a corrective letter to the paper. Letter from President of GAC to Prefect, April 15, 1881, AD, Rhône, 1X2.
49. Deliberations of GAC HCL, January 25, 1882.
50. *Croisure* at Croix-Rousse Hospital, Deliberations of GAC HCL, April 8, 1883.
51. See Timothy B. Smith, "Republicans, Catholics and Social Reform: Lyon, 1870–1920," *French History,* 12 (1998): 1–30, esp. 12–18.
52. The religious orders were able surreptitiously to buy back a portion of their properties, and after 1885 had reestablished themselves in Lyons. Some of the teaching orders masqueraded as lay instructors to avoid censure. Latreille, "La Vie politique et le mouvement des idées," p. 359.
53. "Les Infirmières des hospices de Lyon," *RP* (August 10, 1901): 465–466; *Procès-verbaux du Conseil Municipal de Lyon,* May 15, 1880.
54. *Procès-verbaux du Conseil Municipal de Lyon,* February 15, 1881; October 6, 1881.
55. *Procès-verbaux du Conseil Municipal de Lyon,* February 12, 1884. A strong minority on the council backed a version of the resolution that called for the radical laicization of all nursing staffs in the HCL.
56. Ibid.
57. Ibid.
58. Ibid.
59. Deliberations of GAC HCL, November 18, 1885.
60. *Procès-verbaux du Conseil Municipal de Lyon,* May 21, 1887. On Emile Combes' efforts to have religious symbols removed from public institutions, see Gérard Cholvy and Yves-Marie Hilaire, *Histoire religieuse de la France contemporaine, 1880/1930* (Toulouse: Privat, 1986) p. 105.
61. Deliberations of GAC HCL, May 15, 1912.
62. Deliberations of GAC HCL, April 23, 1920.
63. In Lyons, socialism achieved unprecedented popularity in working class neighborhoods like Brotteaux and the Croix-Rousse, where many of the hospitals' patients resided.

64. Letter, April 20, 1905, AD, Rhône 1X2.

65. Letter from patients to mayor, November 26, 1901, and letter/report from bursar of Croix-Rousse to President of GAC, December 20, 1901, AD, Rhône, 1X2.

66. Letter dated October 5, 1905, AD, Rhône, 1X2.

67. Letter and inquiry from Perron Hospice to Deputé, January 22, 1909, AD, Rhône, 1X2.

68. Letters, undated, March-April 1910, AD, Rhône, 1X2.

69. Caillemer, *croisure* at Saint-Pothin Hospital, May 9, 1909, *Discours*, p. 32.

70. Caillemer, *croisure* at Perron Hospice, May 19, 1912, *Discours*, p. 62.

71. For a discussion of the reception of the law separating Church and state in Lyons, primarily according to the city's daily press, see Laperrière, *La "Séparation" à Lyon (1904–1908)*.

72. *Procès-verbaux du Conseil Municipal de Lyon*, January 28, 1896, p. 226; *L'Organisation spéciale des hospices civils de Lyon* (Lyons, 1913).

73. Paul-Louis Lande, "L'Organisation des hôpitaux de province," in *Conseil international des nurses (gardes-malades), Conférence du Nursing, La troisième séance de tous congrès internationaux des nurses, Paris, June 18–22, 1907*, p. 41; see also *L'Organisation spéciale des Hospices Civils de Lyon*, which notes that city commissions typically had seven members: the mayor, two muncipal council members, and four prefectural nominees.

74. For a detailed description of the patrimony and finances of the Hospices Civils de Lyons, see Maurice Garden, "Le Patrimoine immobilier des Hospices Civils de Lyon, 1800–1914," *Cahiers d'histoire: Lyon, Grenoble, Clermont, Saint-Etienne, Chambéry*, 29 (1984): 119–134.

75. Maurice Rochaix, *Essai sur l'évolution des questions hospitalières de la fin de l'Ancien Régime à nos jours* (Fédération hospitalière de France, 1959), quoted in Garden, "Le Patrimoine immobilier," pp. 119–120.

76. Garden, "Le Patrimoine immobilier," p. 134.

77. Deliberations of GAC HCL, January 12, 1910.

78. Caillemer, *Les Hospices Civils de Lyon*, Conférence à la Société d'Economie Politique et d'Economie Sociale de Lyon, 26 March 1909 (Lyons, 1909), p. 62.

79. Caillemer, *croisure* at Perron, May 19, 1912, *Discours*, p. 60.

80. See Martha L. Hildreth, *Doctors, Bureaucrats and Public Health in France, 1888–1902* (New York: Garland, 1987); Jack D. Ellis, *The Physician-Legislators of France: Medicine and Politics in the Early Third Republic, 1870–1914* (Cambridge: Cambridge University Press, 1990).

81. Victor Augagneur, "L'Instruction technique du personnel hospitalier," *Province médicale*, 3 (April 6, 1889): 159–160.

82. The law of 20 June 1920, which gave the municipal council ten seats on the GAC and reduced the prefect's selections to twenty, made no mention of

medical representation, and only five of the thirty GAC members had medical credentials, a far cry from Augagneur's goal of fifty percent. Report on Hospices Civils de Lyon, 1909, AM, Lyons; *Comptes-morales administratifs des Hospices Civils de Lyon*, 1906, 1916, 1920; Lande, "L'Organisation des hôpitaux de province," p. 41; *Province médicale*, 4 (January 19, 1889): 28.

83. Deliberations of GAC HCL, March 20, 1912.

84. *Croisure* at the Hôtel-Dieu, July 29, 1895, July 24, 1889, Deliberations of GAC HCL.

85. Croze, *Les Soeurs hospitalières des Hospices Civils de Lyon*, p. 118.

86. *Province médicale*, April 6, 1889.

87. *Lyon médical*, 52 (December 28, 1890).

88. Deliberations of GAC HCL, September 20, 1899.

89. Dr. Maurice Letulle, "Rapport présenté au nom de la commission spéciale, Programme de l'enseignement professionnel pour les écoles d'infirmiers et d'infirmières, 1899," CSAP, fascicule 69, p. 5.

90. Letulle, "Rapport présenté au nom de la commission spéciale," p. 6; Faivre, "Rapport présenté au nom de la IIe section, Programme de l'enseignement professionnel pour les écoles d'infirmiers et d'infirmières," 1899, CSAP, fascicule 69, p. 9.

91. Faivre, "Rapport présenté au nom de la IIe section," pp. 8–9.

92. Dozens of *croisure* speeches invoke this theme. The term "demi-savantes" appears for the first time in Sabran's speech at the Hôtel-Dieu on March 25, 1903. Deliberations of GAC HCL, March 25, 1903.

93. *Croisure* at Croix-Rousse Hospital, April 29, 1900, Deliberation of GAC HCL. Sabran delivered the same warning at the *croisure* ceremony at la Charité, December 14, 1901.

94. "Hospices Civils de Lyon: Ecole d'Infirmières, Note sur son fonctionnement," [1904], AM, Lyons, Q3. The document most probably originated with the GAC and was sent to the municipal council.

95. Deliberations of GAC HCL, November 8, 1899.

96. *L'Assistance publique*, 22 (November 30, 1900): 315.

97. *Procès-verbaux du Conseil Municipal*, November 20, 1900.

98. The GAC recognized that without offering financial assistance, it could not hope to attract "civilian" young women to the school or the profession. Accordingly, by the beginning of the 1901–1902 school year, the Departmental Council of the Rhône created four scholarships, and the GAC agreed to support three or four students each year. The HCL's financial status became increasingly precarious as the century progressed, however, and by October 1914 the administration no longer offered financial support. *RP*, 9 (September 10, 1901): 582; *Lyon médical*, 39 (September 29, 1901): 458; undated note in "Ecole" folder, HCL Archives.

99. *RP,* 9 (September 10, 1901): 582; Letter from Prefect of Rhône to President of GAC, January 13, 1910, HCL Archives; "Hospices Civils de Lyon, Ecole d'Infirmières; Note sur son fonctionnement," [1904], AM, Lyons, Q3. In Lyons, most home nursing care was provided by religious congregations such as the Filles de la Charité de Saint Vincent de Paul.

100. Letters dated February 26, 1910 and April 7, 1905, HCL Archives, box labeled "Ecole d'infirmières."

101. Correspondence between Prefect of Drôme, Prefect of Rhône, and President of GAC and letter from President of GAC to Prefect of Rhône, dated September 10, 1904, in HCL Archives, box labeled "Ecole d'infirmières."

102. *Lyon médical,* 18 (September 25, 1920): 802.

103. Document dated February 5, 1914, HCL Archives, box labeled "Soeurs hospitalières, Conditions d'admission à l'Ecole d'Infirmières, 1887, 1911–14"; Deliberations of GAC HCL, *croisure* at Hôtel-Dieu, July 24, 1889.

104. Letter from Prefect to President du Conseil, Ministre de l'Intérieur et des Cultes, dated June 10, 1910, in AD, Rhône, 1Xp 228.

105. Deliberations of GAC HCL, November 8, 1911; "Listes des elèves, Ecole d'Infirmières, années 1911–1912, 1912–1913," HCL Archives, box labeled "Ecole d'infirmières"; Deliberations of GAC HCL, October 6, 1915.

106. Letter from Prefect to President du Conseil, Ministre de l'Intérieur et des Cultes, dated June 10, 1910, in AD, Rhône, 1Xp 228.

107. Specifically, he wanted to replace conservative GAC members with men who supported Herriot's plan to tear down the Hôtel-Dieu and construct a modern hospital on the outskirts of the city.

108. Untitled document, February 5, 1914, HCL Archives, box labeled "Soeurs hospitalières, Conditions d'admission à l'Ecole d'Infirmières, 1887, 1911–14."

109. Deliberations of GAC HCL, October 18, 1916.

110. Letter from Director of Charité to GAC, in Deliberations of GAC HCL, May 2, 1917.

111. Deliberations of GAC HCL, May 31, 1899.

112. Deliberations of GAC HCL, March 29, 1905. Called *veilleuses,* the women on night-duty were usually untrained and worked for paltry hourly wages. Reformers in Paris, Lyons, and Bordeaux all recognized the need to integrate night-duty into standard training for the nursing diploma. Only in Bordeaux, however, was this recognition translated into policy.

113. Caillemer, *croisure* at the Hôtel-Dieu, January 24, 1912, *Discours,* p. 57.

114. *Compte moral administratif,* 1912, 1916, and 1922.

115. "Règlement pour les communautés de tous les établissements," February 14, 1939, HCL Archives, box labeled "Personnel hospitalier, Frères et Soeurs, Règlementations."

3. The *Gardes-malades* of Bordeaux

1. *AJN*, 8 (December 1907): 203. See also Paul-Louis Lande, "La Question des infirmières," *Journal de médecine de Bordeaux*, 43 (October 23, 1904): 768.

2. Published in Paris, this more popularized version was co-edited with Félix Regnault, a former Paris intern and former doctor at the Hôtel-Dieu in Marseille. The entire volume has been reprinted in *Soins*, 22 (August 5 and 20, 1977): 81–88; (December 5, 1977): 43–51; (December 20, 1977): 45–50; and *Soins*, 23 (April 20, 1978): 21–28.

3. Anna-Emilie Hamilton, "Considérations sur les infirmières des hôpitaux," MD thesis, Faculté de medécine de Montpellier, 1900, pp. 122, 125.

4. Letter from Hamilton to Lavinia Dock, December 29, 1907, Adelaide Nutting Papers, Teachers College, Columbia University, Nutting Collection, microfiche 2442.

5. Letter from Hamilton to Lavinia Dock, April 3, 1910, Nutting Collection, microfiche 2013. For a detailed description of Anna Hamilton's youth and education, including citations from a journal revised by Hamilton later in her life, see Evelyne Diebolt, *La Maison de Santé Protestante de Bordeaux (1863–1934)* (Toulouse: Erès, 1990), pp. 45–51. See also Marguerite Fechner, "A Montpellier une étudiante de jadis Anna Hamilton, 1864–1935," *Bulletin historique de la Ville de Montpellier*, 11 (1985): 5–8, in Bibliothèque Marguerite Durand, file "Hamilton."

6. The copy of "Considérations" in the Archives of the Assistance Publique in Paris contains a handwritten page taped in the book entitled "Journée de la religieuse." According to the unnamed author of the account, the religious sister limited her nursing duties to serving meals and following the attending physician's rounds. A significant portion of the day was spent in prayer and by early evening she had retired for the day. It is unclear why this sheet was added to the book. The handwriting does not resemble Hamilton's.

7. Hamilton, "Considérations," p. 55.

8. Ibid., p. 91.

9. For a theoretical discussion of the roots of nursing in religion and specifically Catholicism, see Marie-Françoise Collière, *Promouvoir la vie* (Paris: Inter-éditions, 1982), pp. 49–74.

10. Hamilton, "Considérations," p. 144.

11. A similar argument had already been made by the special committee of the national Conseil Supérieur de l'Assistance Publique appointed by the Minister of the Interior to establish national guidelines for the development of nursing schools throughout the country. Faivre, "Rapport présenté au nom de la IIe section, Programme de l'enseignement professionnel pour les écoles d'infirmiers et d'infirmières," 1899, CSAP, fascicule 69, p. 12. See also Dr.

Henri Napias, "Recrutement du personnel secondaire des établissements hospitaliers," CSAP, fascicule 69.

12. Hamilton, "Considérations," p. 129.

13. Hamilton noted that a single school in the Department of the Seine received 8,014 requests for employment by the end of 1898, and an estimated 15,000 to 20,000 were waiting for jobs in banks and shops. "Considérations," pp. 292–293; Jo Burr Margadant writes that the young women trained as teachers at the Ecole de Sèvres could no longer count on permanent employment after 1890 as a result of a severe slowdown in the creation of secondary schools for girls; *Madame le Professeur, Women Educators in the Third Republic* (Princeton: Princeton University Press, 1990), pp. 100–101.

14. Hamilton, "Considérations," p. 129.

15. Lavinia L. Dock, "The Bordeaux Schools of Nursing," *AJN*, 8 (December 1907): 202.

16. Dr. Julien Noir, "Procès-verbal des prix distribués à l'école d'infirmiers et infirmières de Bicêtre, 1904–5," in AAP, Fosseyeux 646, vol. 34.

17. Hamilton, "Considérations," p. 127.

18. Martha Vicinus, *Independent Women: Work and Community for Single Women, 1850–1920* (Chicago: University of Chicago Press, 1985), p. 89. Vicinus argues that from about 1840 to 1890 women who joined religious sisterhoods were able to break out of the restrictive role assigned them as members of the Victorian middle class by taking on full-time work in the slums and hospitals. Vicinus stresses that although these women defied social norms, their morality-driven work among the poor, sick, and "fallen" also served to highlight and strengthen class differences.

19. Hamilton, "Considérations," p. 273.

20. Ibid., pp. 275–276.

21. Ibid., p. 152. Similar restrictions on marriage applied to the lay women teachers introduced after the 1880 reforms in girls' education. By the 1890s, however, the difficulty of retaining female teachers in rural areas forced the government to reverse its policy on celibacy. See Leslie Page Moch, "Government Policy and Women's Experience: The Case of Teachers in France," *Feminist Studies*, 14 (Summer 1988): 301–324. On the expectation that secular teachers would behave like nuns, see Judith Wishnia, *The Proletarianizing of the Fonctionnaires: Civil Service Workers and the Labor Movement under the Third Republic* (Baton Rouge: Louisiana State University Press, 1990), p. 50.

22. Hamilton, "Considérations," p. 280.

23. Ibid., pp. ix–x.

24. Ibid., p. 285.

25. *GM* (June 1907): 133.

26. Hamilton's letters to nursing leaders in the United States are filled with tales

of the seduction of young nurses by salacious interns and doctors and of the wanton behavior of Red Cross "lady nurses." Her strict standards for "moral behavior" appear to be more idiosyncratic than endemic to the Bordeaux reform movement, although a concern for unimpeachable conduct was part of the general effort to distinguish nursing from domestic service.

27. For a provocative discussion of the class basis of Florence Nightingale's reforms, see Mary Poovey, *Uneven Developments: The Ideological Work of Gender in Mid-Victorian England* (Chicago: University of Chicago Press, 1988), pp. 164–201.

28. Anna Hamilton and Felix Régnault, *Les Gardes-malades: Congréganistes, mercenaires, amateurs, professionnelles* (Paris, 1901), reprinted in *Soins*, 23 (April 1978): 25.

29. Anne Summers explores the close connection between skills used by middle-class women in managing large household staffs to those required to manage a nursing corps in British military hospitals, in *Angels and Citizens: British Women as Military Nurses, 1854–1914* (London: Routledge and Kegan Paul, 1988). Jo Burr Margadant makes a similar observation about the Ecole de Sèvres in *Madame le Professeur*, esp. p. 40. See also Poovey, *Uneven Developments*, pp. 191–193.

30. Lande was elected mayor in 1900 as part of the left-republican list that ousted the bizarre Pacte de Bordeaux—an anti-Opportunist left-right coalition—from power. Among his numerous public and professional roles, Lande was a founding member of the Union des Syndicats Médicaux de France and served as its president during the 1880s. In 1911 he became the first non-Parisian to hold the presidency of the powerful Association Générale des Médecins de France. *GM* (May 1912): 65–109. See also Lande's obituary in *La France du Sud-Ouest*, April 24, 1912.

31. Maison de Santé Protestante, 23ème Rapport annuel, 1884, pp. 11–12, in AD, Gironde, 1N454; *Notice sur la Maison de Santé Protestante* (Bordeaux, 1891), p. 27, in AM, Bordeaux, 660Q1. See also Diebolt, *La Maison de Santé Protestante*, p. 41.

32. *Ecole Florence Nightingale cinquentenaire* (Bordeaux, 1934), p. 9.

33. Letter from Hamilton to Lavinia L. Dock, Nov. 5, 1906, Nutting Collection, microfiche no. 2442.

34. From a high of 150 in 1884–85, student attendance dropped to 35 in 1889–90. *Notice sur la Maison de Santé Protestante de Bordeaux*, p. 27; Maison de Santé Protestante, Rapport annuel, 1884, p. 33. See also "Dans les hôpitaux," *BP*, 13 (April 15, 1905): 43.

35. *PM* (January 19, 1895): 42–43.

36. *PM* (October 19, 1895): 247.

37. Gabriel Faure appointed her to the position of *médecin résident* in 1900.

When Mme. Momméja resigned in November 1901, Hamilton became *directrice* of all the Maison's services, including the school. Anna Hamilton, "Les Ecoles hospitalières de gardes-malades de Bordeaux," in *Conseil international des nurses (gardes-malades), Conférence du Nursing, La troisième séance de tous congrès internationaux des nurses, Paris, 18–22 June 1907* (Bordeaux: Imprimerie commerciale et industrielle, 1907), p. 48.

38. Hamilton, *Plan pour les cours théoriques d'une école hospitalière de gardes-malades Florence Nightingale* (Bordeaux, s.d.).

39. Hamilton, "Les Ecoles hospitalières," *Conseil international des nurses (1907)*, pp. 56–60.

40. Ibid., p. 48.

41. *Ecole Florence Nightingale cinquantenaire*, p. 23.

42. Hamilton, "Les Ecoles hospitalières," *Conseil international des nurses (1907)*, p. 48.

43. "Extrait du rapport de la Directrice, compte rendu de la Maison de Santé Protestante, 1906," reprinted in *GM* (January 1910): 29.

44. Hamilton, "Les Ecoles hospitalières," *Conseil international des nurses (1907)*, p. 51.

45. Ibid., p. 60.

46. *AJN*, 6 (February 1906): 316.

47. "Dans les hôpitaux," *BP*, 13 (April 1905): 43. The ten departments listed were: Aveyron, Drôme, Indre-et-Loire, Gironde, Basses-Pyrennées, Côte-d'Or, Dordogne, Ardêche, Vosges, and Seine.

48. *GM* (March 1909): 55.

49. Statistics from *GM*, 1906–1912; Hamilton, "Les Ecoles hospitalières," *Conseil international des nurses (1907)*; *RP*, 37 (August 15, 1916): 366.

50. *GM* (March 1912): 48.

51. *GM* (June 1911): 117. Upon her death in 1914, Elisabeth Bosc, a 1906 graduate who served as *cheftaine* in the Alès Hospital and as *directrice* in St.-Quentin, donated to the school a large tract of land in Bagatelle, outside the city. After the war, the MSP, together with the renamed Ecole Florence Nightingale, moved to Bagatelle with the financial assistance of the Seltzer family, three of whose daughters graduated from the Bordeaux schools. Fechner, "A Montpellier une étudiante de jadis," p. 8.

52. *GM* (September 1906): 29; (November 1906): 45; (January 1907): 60; (May 1907): 27; (March 1909): 42.

53. Hamilton, "Les Ecoles hospitalières," *Conseil international des nurses (1907)*, p. 63; *BP*, 13 (April 15, 1905): 43; *GM* (April 1909): 71; (May 1910): 110; (September 1910): 194–195; (March 1912): 47.

54. Administrators often compared these salaries to the 200-franc stipend granted most nursing sisters and found the Bordeaux scheme extravagant

and unjustifiable. Hamilton, Lande, and other promoters of the schools insisted that because the *gardes-malades* performed patient care as well as supervisory functions, the Bordeaux system required fewer nurses and was, as a result, only slightly more expensive.

55. Lavinia L. Dock, "French Provincial Hospitals," *AJN*, 8 (February 1908): 388. Cumulative statistics from *GM*, 1906–1914; *Conseil international des nurses (1907)*.

56. *GM* (July 1906): 16; (March 1907): 95; (July 1910): 46; (October 1911): 61. *BP* (April 1905); *GM* (July 1906): 16; (January 1907): 60–61; (March 1907): 95; (July 1911): 139.

57. Marguérite Fechner, "Mademoiselle," *Le Sud-Ouest,* 1985, in Bibliothèque Marguerite Durand, file "Hamilton."

58. *Procès-verbaux de la Commission Administrative des Hospices de Bordeaux,* November 21, 1902, AD, Gironde, 5M582.

59. Letter from Lande to Prefect Charles Lutaud, July 10, 1903, AD, Gironde, 5M582; Letter from Prefect Charles Lutaud to Lande, August 15, 1903, AD, Gironde, 5M582.

60. AD, Gironde, 5M582; *La France,* October 24, 1903; October 31, 1903.

61. *La Nouvelliste,* November 1903.

62. J.-M. Durand, "Instruction professionnelle et situation du personnel secondaire des hôpitaux," *III Congrès National d'Assistance Publique et de Bienfaisance Privée, troisième question du Congrès* (Bordeaux: Imprimerie G. Gounouilhou, 1903) p. 13.

63. Dr. Charles Mongour, *Rapport sur l'utilité de la création à l'Hôpital Saint-André d'une école d'infirmiers et d'infirmières* (Bordeaux, 1900), p. 3.

64. AD, Gironde, 5M582, especially letter from Hospital Administrative Commission to Prefect of the Gironde, November 27, 1902.

65. X. Arnozan, "La Question des infirmières," *Journal de médecine de Bordeaux,* 46 (November 15, 1903): 741–742.

66. *Journal de médecine de Bordeaux,* 50 (December 13, 1903): 815; 49 (December 6, 1903): 795.

67. "Inauguration de l'Ecole de gardes-malades de Bordeaux," *PM,* 19 (February 27, 1904): 137.

68. Extrait du Registre des Délibérations de la HAC, April 8, 1904, in AD, Gironde, 5M582.

69. *La Nouvelliste,* February 2, 1904, reprinted in *La Croix,* February 3, 1904.

70. Letter from the Prefect of the Gironde to President of the Conseil Ministériel de l'Intérieur et des Cultes, January 2, 1905, AD, Gironde, 5M582. Daney had already served two terms as mayor of Bordeaux, from 1884 to 1888 and from 1892 to 1896. In 1904 he ran on a list composed heavily of nationalists, and whose slogan was "neither reaction, nor revolution." L. Desgraves and G.

Dupeux, eds., *Bordeaux au XIXe siècle* (Bordeaux: Fédération historique du Sud-Ouest, 1969), pp. 323–345.

71. Letter from the Prefect of the Gironde to the President of the Conseil Ministériel de l'Intérieur et des Cultes, January 2, 1905, AD, Gironde, 5M582.

72. Ironically, Arnozan had himself suggested that Lande establish the school for "nurses à la mode anglaise," in Tondu in November 1903, in an attempt to keep the new school out of Saint-André. *Journal de médecine de Bordeaux*, 46 (November 15, 1903): 741.

73. AD, Gironde, 5M582, *Procès-verbaux de la Commission Administrative des Hospices de Bordeaux*, November 21, 1902.

74. "'Nurses' francaises. Bordeaux possède le modèle des écoles d'infirmières laiques," *Le Matin*, August 25, 1906.

75. *Ecole de Gardes-malades Hospitalières de l'Hôpital Civil du Tondu, Bordeaux* (s.l.n.d)[1909], p. 26.

76. *GM* (December 1907): 236–237.

77. Ibid., p. 236.

78. Ibid.

79. *GM* (March 1911): 37–38.

80. Ibid., p. 41.

81. Catherine Elston, "Retour de Lorient," *GM* (February 1911): 21.

82. Letter from Hamilton to Lavinia Dock, May 30, 1911, Nutting Collection, microfiche 2442.

83. Elston, "Retour de Lorient," p. 37.

84. Lavinia L. Dock, "French Provincial Hospitals," *AJN*, 8 (February 1908): 389.

85. Letter from Mirman, Direction de l'Assistance et Hygiène Publique, Ministère de l'Intérieur, to Prefect of the Gironde, May 1, 1912. AD, Gironde, Archives of Tondu Hospital, uncatalogued.

86. Letter from the Commission Administrative des Hospices de Bordeaux to Prefect, May 4, 1912. AD, Gironde, Archives of Tondu Hospital, uncatalogued.

87. *Bordeaux au XIXe siècle*, pp. 368–369.

88. Pastoral letter from Cardinal-Archbishop of Bordeaux, on the occasion of his arrival in his diocese, *L'Aquitaine*, April 2, 1909, quoted in *Bordeaux au XIXe siècle*, p. 369.

89. Charles Cazalet, "Rapport présenté le 4 October 1912 à la Commission des Hospices Civils de Bordeaux sur l'Hôpital du Tondu et l'Ecole de Gardes-malades laiques," p. 10, AD, Gironde, Archives of Tondu Hospital, uncatalogued.

90. *GM*, 69 (June 1912): 111–112.

91. Letter from Hamilton to Adelaide Nutting, July 10, 1920, Nutting Collection, microfiche 2495.

92. Nonetheless, in the short decade and a half before the First World War, grad-

uates of both the Tondu school and the MSP accepted directorships in nine hospitals and were sent to reorganize the nursing staffs in the principal municipal hospitals of eight cities. Cazalet, "Rapport présenté le 4 Octobre 1912," p. 24.

93. Diebolt, *La Maison de Santé Protestante,* pp. 118–120.

94. *La Française,* February 21, 1914.

95. *GM,* 69 (June 1912): 113.

4. Class, Gender, and Professional Identity

1. See especially Barbara Melosh, *"The Physician's Hand": Work Culture and Conflict in American Nursing* (Philadelphia: University of Pennsylvania Press, 1982), pp. 15–29. See also Gerald L. Geison, ed., *Professions and the French State, 1700–1900* (Philadelphia: Temple University Press, 1984). For a classic analysis of professionalization as applied to medicine, see Eliot Freidson, *Profession of Medicine: A Study of the Sociology of Applied Knowledge* (New York: Harper and Row, 1970).

2. "L'Ecole des Infirmières de l'Assistance Publique," *BP* (June 15, 1908): 61–62.

3. Ministère du Travail et de la Prévoyance Sociale, *Annuaire des syndicats professionnels, industriels, commerciaux et agricoles,* 19 vols. (Paris: Imprimerie nationale, 1896–1914). The statistics and analysis presented in this chapter do not include organizations of mental asylum personnel. Catherine Smet has identified 45 professional organizations of hospital workers, including mental asylum employees. Smet, "Secularization and Syndicalization: The Rise of Professional Nursing in France, 1870–1914," Ph.D. diss., University of California, San Diego, 1997, pp. 185–235.

4. Melosh, *"The Physician's Hand,"* p. 5.

5. Significantly, although unhappily from the point of view of the historian, none of the hospital employees organizations made a distinction between those who worked with patients and those who supervised nonmedical services like food preparation or laundry. Except where otherwise noted, then, the term "nurses" should be understood as a direct translation of the vague titles "infirmier" and "infirmière."

6. Administrative representatives frequently referred to the employees, administration, doctors, and patients of public hospitals as the "great hospital family." Nurses were often cast as older children, at once responsible for their helpless younger siblings (the patients) and subordinate to their parents (the administration and/or doctors). See, for example, *Voix du Peuple,* November 14, 1909.

7. Note from Secretariat Général de l'Assistance Publique, May 3, 1902, AAP, Fosseyeux 618, box 1. On the development of syndicalism and socialism, see

Judith F. Stone, *The Search for Social Peace: Reform Legislation in France, 1890–1914* (Albany: State University of New York Press, 1985), pp. 83–96; Kathryn E. Amdur, *Syndicalist Legacy: Trade Unions and Politics in Two French Cities in the Era of World War I* (Urbana, Ill.: University of Illinois Press, 1986), pp. 32–55; Jacques Kergoat, "France," in *The Formation of Labour Movements, 1870–1914: An International Perspective,* Marcel van der Linden and Jürgen Rojahn, eds. (Leiden: E. J. Brill, 1990), pp. 163–190; Peter N. Stearns, *Revolutionary Syndicalism and French Labor* (New Brunswick: Rutgers University Press, 1971), pp. 1–33; Theodore Zeldin, *France 1848–1945,* vol. I, *Politics and Anger* (Oxford, New York: Oxford University Press, 1984), pp. 334–346; Judith Wishnia, *The Proletarianizing of the Fonctionnaires: Civil Service Workers and the Labor Movement under the Third Republic* (Baton Rouge: Louisiana State University Press, 1990).

8. "Les Infirmiers et infirmières des hôpitaux et hospices de Bordeaux," *PM,* 23 (August 24, 1907): 541–542.

9. *L'Infirmier,* January 1900, special edition.

10. *BM* (December 1913).

11. *Annuaire des syndicats professionnels,* vol. 10 (1905); vol. 14 (1909); vol. 17 (1912).

12. Huyvetter, "Une Circulaire," *L'Action,* May 1, 1907.

13. These figures include agricultural workers and their syndicates. Madeleine Guilbert, *Les Femmes et l'organisation syndicale avant 1914* (Paris: Editions du Centre National de la Recherche Scientifique, 1966), pp. 29–34. See also Mary Lynn Stewart, *Women, Work, and the French State: Labour Protection and Social Patriarchy, 1879–1919* (Kingston, Ontario: McGill-Queen's University Press, 1989), p. 22. Trade union participation in France was weak for both men and women, representing only 7 percent of the entire labor force in 1911. Louise A. Tilly and Joan W. Scott, *Women, Work and Family* (New York: Methuen, 1987), p. 188. Guilbert puts that figure at 4.5 percent.

14. A growing body of literature focuses on the gendered dimensions of labor history. See, for example, Judith Coffin, "Social Science Meets Sweated Labor: Reinterpreting Women's Work in Late Nineteenth-Century France," *Journal of Modern History,* 63 (June 1991): 230–270; Coffin, "Credit, Consumption, and Images of Women's Desires: Selling the Sewing Machine in Late Nineteenth-Century France," *French Historical Studies,* 18 (Spring 1994): 749–783; Coffin, *The Politics of Women's Work: The Paris Garment Trades, 1750–1915* (Princeton, N.J.: Princeton University Press, 1996); Joan Wallach Scott, *Gender and the Politics of History* (New York: Columbia University Press, 1988), esp. pp. 93–163; and Scott, "The Woman Worker," in Georges Duby and Michelle Perrot, eds., *A History of Women,* vol. 4., *Emerging Feminism from Revolution to World War* (Cambridge, Mass.: Harvard University Press, 1993),

pp. 399–426; Charles Sowerwine, "Workers and Women in France before 1914: The Debate over the Couriau Affair," *Journal of Modern History*, 55 (September 1983): 411–441; Stewart, *Women, Work, and the French State.*

15. Name changes, in some cases frequent, make it difficult to determine precisely how many different organizations were created.

16. *BM* (July–August 1904).

17. A. Filiatre, "Règlement du Syndicat et Union Fraternelle des Sous-Employés et Infirmiers de l'Assistance Publique," November 4, 1891, AAP, Fosseyeux 618, box 1.

18. "Règlement de la Chambre Syndicale des Infirmiers, Infirmières et Garde-malades du Departement de la Seine," 1892, AAP, Fosseyeux 618, box 1.

19. Letters from Coutant to Director AP, December 30, 1892, January 31, 1893, April 1, 1893, AAP, Fosseyeux 618, box 1.

20. Letter from Coutant to AP, December 2, 1892, AAP, Fosseyeux 618, box 1.

21. Letter from Coutant to AP, April 1, 1893, AAP Fosseyeux 618, box 1. The *Radical* reported on December 9, 1892, that the Director of Bicêtre threatened to fire all those who attended syndicate meetings. He angrily denied the allegations, stating that nurses were free to attend meetings outside work hours. Letter from Director of Bicêtre to AP Director, December 9, 1892, AAP, Fosseyeux 618, box 1.

22. *Annuaire des syndicats professionnels*, vol. 1 (1896), vol. 2 (1897), vol. 4 (1899), vol. 5 (1900), vol. 6 (1901), vol. 7 (1902).

23. Letter from Coutant to Director General of AP, April 30, 1902, AAP, Fosseyeux 618, box 1.

24. Ibid.

25. *PM*, 16 (November 26, 1892): 460–461.

26. *Le Temps*, November 18, 1892.

27. "Syndicat d'infirmiers et d'infirmières," *PM*, 17 (January 14, 1893): 45. Unlike Bourneville, who stressed the absolute necessity of the diploma, the syndicate also included experience in the hospitals as a criterion for preferred status.

28. Statuts du Groupement du Personnel Secondaire de l'Assistance Publique, AAP, Fosseyeux 618, box 1.

29. *L'Union des ouvriers municipaux* 1, no. 8 (supplément), (undated, [1901]), AAP, Fosseyeux 618.

30. Statuts du Groupement du Personnel Secondaire de l'Assistance Publique, AAP, Fosseyeux 618, box 1.

31. *L'Infirmier*, June 4, 1899.

32. Ibid.

33. *L'Infirmier*, June 18, 1899. On Socialist and syndicalist attitudes toward women's work, see Sowerwine, "Workers and Women in France before 1914," pp. 413–414; Sowerwine, *Sisters or Citizens? Women and Socialism in France*

since 1876 (Cambridge: Cambridge University Press, 1982); Marilyn Boxer, "Socialism Faces Feminism: The Failure of Synthesis in France, 1879–1914," in Marilyn J. Boxer and Jean H. Quataert, eds., *Socialist Women: European Socialist Feminism in the Nineteenth and Early Twentieth Centuries* (New York: Elsevier, 1978); Joan Wallach Scott, "Work Identities for Men and Women: The Politics of Work and Family in the Parisian Garment Trades in 1848," in *Gender and the Politics of History,* pp. 93–112.

34. *L'Infirmier,* June 25–July 2, 1899. Dubois's position so closely resembles that of L'Héritier that one is left wondering if Dubois was simply a pseudonym for the journal's editor.

35. *L'Infirmier,* January 19, 1900; *La Fronde,* December 31, 1899; *L'Union des ouvriers municipaux* (undated loose issue [1901]), in AAP, Fosseyeux 618.

36. *La Fronde,* December 31, 1899; *L'Infirmier,* édition speciale(undated [January 1900]).

37. *L'Union des ouvriers municipaux* 1, no. 8 (supplément) (undated [1901]), in AAP, Fosseyeux 618.

38. *L'Infirmier,* édition spéciale (undated [January 1900]).

39. Letter from Artreux to Director of AP, March 25, 1901, in *L'Union des ouvriers municipaux* (undated [April 1901]), AAP, Fosseyeux 618; *BM* (May 1909). Percentages are based on total "secondary staff" statistics from Ministère du Commerce, de l'Industrie, des Postes et des Telegraphs, Direction du Travail, *Statistique générale de la France, Statistique annuelle des institutions d'assistance,* 1899, 1900 (Paris: Imprimerie nationale, 1902).

40. Letter from Artreux to Director of AP, March 25, 1901, *L'Union des ouvriers municipaux* (undated [April 1901]), AAP, Fosseyeux 618.

41. *L'Union des ouvriers municipaux* (undated [April 1901]), AAP, Fosseyeux 618.

42. Letter from L'Héritier to Director of AP, April 10, 1901, in *L'Union des ouvriers municipaux* (undated [April 1901]), AAP, Fosseyeux 618.

43. *L'Union des ouvriers municipaux* (undated [April 1901]), AAP, Fosseyeux 618.

44. *L'Infirmier,* January 22, 1899.

45. The administration justified the rejection by invoking the 1884 law on syndicates which, the AP noted, pertained only to industrial, commercial, and agricultural workers. Letter dated June 12, 1901, from Prefect of the Seine to Waldeck-Rousseau, reprinted in *L'Aurore,* [June 1901], in AAP, Fosseyeux 618, clipping file.

46. *BP,* 13 (April 15, 1905): 46.

47. The SPNG retained the Syndicat du Personnel Secondaire's original syndicate number 1574. "Association et Syndicat," *BM* (May 1909); "Revendications du Syndicat du Personnel Non-gradé de l'Assistance Publique" [1904], AAP, Fosseyeux 618, box 1.

48. *BM* (April 1905); (February 1906); (January 1907); (May 1909).

49. *BM* (January 1906); (February 1907).

50. *BM* (May 1908).

51. *BM* (April 1906).

52. *BM* (December 1904).

53. *BM* (July–August 1904).

54. *BM* (December 1904).

55. *BM* (July–August 1904).

56. "Philanthropie vraie," *BM* (October 1909).

57. "Relèvement moral!" *BM* (May 1909).

58. A. Mage, "Tout le Monde sur le pont!" *BM* (May 1905).

59. *BM* (January 1906).

60. This awareness of the women's importance to the SASS cause was reflected, to a degree, in the organization itself. While women were underrepresented on the SASS governing council (as they were in almost all labor unions), they were quite visible at gatherings within the individual hospitals. In fact, it was not unusual for local meetings to be run exclusively by *surveillantes*. Their more prominent presence at the smaller gatherings suggests that, despite their general absence from the recorded minutes of meetings, women played an important role in organizing the union locals. *BM* (December 1910); (January–February 1911); (September 1906); (January 1907).

61. "Un Souhait?" *BM* (March 1907).

62. *BM* (March 1907).

63. "Assemblée générale extraordinaire, April 17, 1906," in *BM* (April 1906).

64. AAP, Fosseyeux 603 (94); *L'Hospitalier*, August 1, 1917; "Assemblée générale extraordinaire de la SASS, May 13, 1909," *BM* (May 1909); "Mise au point," *BM* (May 1909).

65. "Revendications du Syndicat du Personnel Non-gradé," *Paris journal*, February 15, 1909; *BM* (March 1913).

66. *L'Action*, March 1905.

67. *Le Petit Journal*, September 12, 1908; *La Petite République*, September 12, 1908.

68. *Le Journal*, December 15, 1912, in AN F[7] 13813; Police notes dated March 18, 1907; March 19, 1907; March 22, 1907; September 8, 1908; November 27, 1909; December 11, 1909; October 24, 1913, AN F[7] 13813.

69. Anonymous AP notes dated July 18, 1906, September 8, 1908, AAP, Fosseyeux 618, box 1; *L'Action*, March 1, 1911.

70. Letter from F. Merma to the editor of *Le Temps*, September 1, 1911, AN F[7] 13814.

71. *L'Ouvrier sanitaire*, June 15, 1910; *Paris journal*, February 15, 1909. Revendications du Syndicat du Personnel Non-Gradé, October 23, 1906 (sent to AP administration, Conseil de Surveillance de l'Assistance Publique, and the Paris Municipal Council), AAP, Fosseyeux 618.

72. Letter from Huyvetter to Director of AP, April 11, 1907, AAP, Fosseyeux 618, box 1.

73. Ibid.

74. Note from AP Director to hospital directors, April 23, 1907, AAP, Fosseyeux 618; anonymous note, August 31, 1908, AAP, Fosseyeux 618; notes dated September 8, 1908, September 11, 1908, AAP, Fosseyeux 618; *La Petite Republique,* September 12, 1908.

75. Administration générale de l'Assistance Publique à Paris, *Projet de réforme du règlement du 1er mai 1903 sur le personnel hospitalier* (Montévrain: Imprimerie de l'Ecole d'Alembert, 1909), pp. 3–8.

76. *Projet de réforme du règlement du 1er mai 1903,* pp. 3–5.

77. Ibid., pp. 5–6.

78. For the *personnel gradé,* the regulation maintained equal salaries for male and female surveillants, but instituted a 50FF differential for the rank of *suppléante.* "Règlement pour le personnel hospitalier, arrêté des 25 mars–19 mai 1910," in AAP, C-2394[4].

79. *Projet de réforme du règlement du 1er mai 1903,* p. 4.

80. The male employees of the Sainte Anne Asylum and Villejuif Hospice lodged a formal complaint against the growing presence of female nurses and *surveillantes* in the male wards, calling the situation "contrary to the morale, the spirit of devotion, and discipline." *L'Action,* December 8, 1909; "L'Egalité pour tous," *L'Action,* July 1, 1910; see also, *Fédération des Services de Santé de France et des Colonies. Ve Congrès Corporatif, 1912* (Bourges: Imprimerie ouvrier du centre ouvriers, syndiqués, et fédérés, 1913).

81. "Simple vérité," *L'Echo des garçons de service de l'Assistance Publique,* August 1, 1910. *L'Echo du personnel hospitalier de l'Assistance Publique,* January 1, 1911. By 1911, the Association admitted women but maintained its policy of separate lists of demands for men and women.

82. Police notes on Assemblée générale trimestrielle of SPNG, April 13, 1910, May 7, 1910, AN F[7] 13813, dossier 2.

83. Police notes dated November 27, 1909, AN F[7] 13813.

84. "Mise au point," *L'Action,* March 1, 1911. Similar arguments were advanced by members of the central committee of the National Federation of Printers' Unions who supported the entry of women into the trade as long as they received equal pay. See Guilbert, *Les Femmes et l'organisation syndicale avant 1914,* pp. 49–64.

85. "Travail égal, pain égal," *Ouvrier sanitaire,* June 15, 1910.

86. Police report dated May 7, 1910, AN F[7] 13813, dossier 2. Police reports from numerous SPNG meetings and demonstrations between late 1909 and 1911 note the singing of the "Internationale."

87. *La Bataille syndicaliste,* June 28, 1911; *La Médecine sociale* (December 1910).

88. Note from AP Director to President of Municipal Council, 5th Commission,

November 16, 1911; Letter from Director of AP to Prefect of Seine, January 1912; Letter from Merma to Director of AP, March 9, 1914; Letters from Director of AP Personnel to Merma, May 20, 1913; March 12, 1914, all in AAP, Fosseyeux 618, box 1.

89. *L'Action,* September 15, 1908; Revendications du personnel non-gradé de l'Assistance Publique, AAP, Fosseyeux 618, box 1.

90. *L'Action,* June 23, 1908; Open letter from Abadie of SPNG to Director-General of AP, *L'Action,* November 15, 1908; September 15, 1908.

91. Several of the cases presented by the SPNG to the administration for consideration for promotions were signed with an "X," indicating complete illiteracy, or were marked "manque d'instruction." AAP, Fosseyeux 603 (93).

92. *Ouvrier sanitaire,* June 15, 1910.

93. *Fédération des Services de Santé de France et des Colonies, Ve Congrès corporatif, 1912* (Bourges: Imprimerie ouvrier du centre ouvriers, syndiqués, et fédérés, 1912), p. 154.

94. One member objected to the motion on the grounds that it invited an "invasion of intellectuals." Meeting of the Conseil Syndical of SPNG, *L'Action,* August 24, 1908.

95. In 1909, three of the fifteen members came from Paris, the rest from Lyons, Bron (a Lyons suburb and location of the departmental mental asylum), Carcassonne, Toulouse, Toulon, Montpellier, Marseille, Nice, Aise, Auch, Montdeverque, Ville-Evrard. Note entitled "La Situation avant le Congrès," AN F⁷13813, dossier 1.

96. *L'Humanité,* July 12, 1907.

97. *L'Humanité,* July 13, 1907; July 14, 1907. The 1900 legislation proposed to institute the ten-hour work day over a period of four years in all industries that employed men, women, and children. Up until then, different work hours applied to different groups: twelve hours for men, eleven for adult women and adolescents, and ten for children. None of the measures had ever been applied to hospitals, which were not considered industrial workplaces. Stone, *The Search for Social Peace,* pp. 128–134; For a detailed history of the reduction of work hours, see Gary Cross, *A Quest for Time: The Reduction of Work in Britain and France, 1840–1940* (Berkeley: University of California Press, 1989).

98. *Fédération des Services de Santé de France et des Colonies, IIème Congrès corporatif, 1908* (Bourges: Imprimerie ouvrier du centre ouvriers, syndiqués, et fédérés, 1908); *Vème Congrès corporatif, 1912.*

99. In September of 1908, for example, an anonymous administration report described an SPNG plan that would place the entire secondary staff under the exclusive authority of the doctors in the event of a strike. Anonymous report dated September 8, 1908, AAP, Fosseyeux 618, box 1.

100. *Fédération des Services de Santé de France et des Colonies, Vème Congrès corporatif, 1912,* pp. 153–155.

101. In order to qualify for the state license, a nurse had to complete a full two years of training at an accredited nursing school that was affiliated with a hospital. In addition, the candidate had to pass a standardized, juried exam. See Chapter 6.

102. *Midi-Socialiste,* September 4, 1909. After the war, Peillod was elected to the Lyons Municipal Council on the Socialist ticket.

103. *Fédération des Services de Santé de France et des Colonies, Vème Congrès corporatif, 1912,* pp. 138–140.

104. "Rapport sur la laïcisation des hôpitaux, hospices et asiles adoptés par les congrès corporatifs de Toulouse 1909 et de Nice 1911," in AAP, Fosseyeux 618.

105. *Fédération des Services de Santé, Vème Congrès corporatif, 1912; PM,* 23 (August 24, 1907): 541–542.

106. *Fédération des Services de Santé, Vème Congrès corporatif, 1912,* pp. 136–145. Peillod noted that the physicians' syndicates were dominated by private practitioners. He argued that in Lyons, for example, the hospital doctors favored laicization while the private doctors opposed it.

5. The Nursing Profession in World War I

1. "La Guerre et le travail féminin," *RP,* 37 (May 15, 1916): 231, 236.

2. R. Thamin, *Revue des deux mondes* (November–December 1919), quoted in Yvonne Knibiehler, ed., *Cornettes et blouses blanches: Les Infirmières dans la société française, 1880–1980* (Paris: Hachette, 1984), p. 108.

3. Monseigneur Touchet, Bishop of Orléans, *Aux Infirmières de France: Quelques Pensées* (Paris, 1916). See Margaret H. Darrow, "French Volunteer Nursing and the Myth of War Experience in World War I," *American Historical Review,* 101 (February 1996): 81–84.

4. Darrow, "French Volunteer Nursing," p. 84.

5. This tendency reflects the types of sources that are readily available: evocative memoirs and diaries, journalistic, autobiographical articles, and the prodigious publications of the three French Red Cross societies.

6. Yvonne Pitrois, *Infirmières héroïques: Les Femmes de 1914–1918,* vol. 2 (Geneva: J. H. Jeheber, n.d.), p. 82.

7. Anne Malterre-Barthe, "Nos Anges gardiens, 1914–1918," in Marie-Françoise Collière and Evelyne Diebolt, eds., *Pour une histoire des soins et des professions soignantes,* cahier no. 10 (Paris: AMIEC, 1988), p. 136.

8. Véronique Leroux-Hugon has argued that the confusion between volunteer and professional nurses proved to be "paradoxically positive for the nursing

profession," for in praising the self-sacrificing, patriotic wartime nurse, the public (and the state) recognized the value of amateur and professional nurse alike. Knibiehler, ed., *Cornettes et blouses blanches*, pp. 81–108; Françoise Thébaud, *La Femme au temps de la guerre de 14* (Paris: Stock, 1986), pp. 83–103.

9. Susan Grayzel makes this point for both British and French women in a broad range of wartime roles in *Women's Identities at War: Gender, Motherhood, and Politics in Britain and France during the First World War* (Chapel Hill: University of North Carolina Press, 1999).

10. *PM*, 17 (April 18, 1903): 295.

11. *PM*, 2 (July 13, 1895): 28.

12. *PM*, 17 (April 18, 1903): 295.

13. Dr. Granjux, *Le Caducée* (January 18, 1908): 21–25, quoted in "Au Val-de-Grâce," *GM* (February 1908): 18.

14. Médecin Inspecteur Troussaint, *Une Page de l'histoire du Service de Santé Militaire* (Paris: Imprimerie librairie militaire, 1919), p. 136; See also Heuyer, *Le Service de Santé est-il prêt pour la guerre de demain?* (Paris, 1913), p. 30.

15. "Des Infirmiers," *GH*, 42 (April 10, 1894): 386–387.

16. *PM*, 19 (February 27, 1904): 138; *PM*, 19 (May 21, 1904): 349.

17. Dr. Felix Regnault, "Les Gardes-malades militaires," *BP*, 13 (July 1905): 74–77; Roger Colomb, "Le Rôle de la femme dans l'assistance aux blessés et malades militaires," quoted in Paul-Louis Lande, "La Question des infirmières," *Journal de médecine de Bordeaux*, 43 (October 23, 1904): 770.

18. *Le Matin*, quoted in *BP*, 15 (October 1907): 125.

19. *BP*, 16 (April 1908): 43–44; Emile Gilbert, *Les Infirmières en temps de guerre* (Moulins, 1902), pp. 9, 12.

20. Anna-Emilie Hamilton, "Considérations sur les infirmières des hôpitaux" (Montpellier, 1900), p. 293.

21. Paul-Louis Lande, "Les Infirmières militaires en France," *GM* (November 1908): 178–179.

22. Dr. Letulle, *La Presse médicale* (January 15, 1908), quoted in "Au Val-de-Grâce," *GM* (March 1908): 40. Dr. Granjux, *Le Caducée* (January 18, 1908): 21–25, quoted in "Au Val-de-Grâce," *GM* (February 1908): 17; Paul-Louis Lande, "Au Val-de-Grâce," *GM* (June 1908): 93.

23. Lande, "Au Val-de-Grâce," p. 92; Alfred Mignon, *Le Service de Santé pendant la guerre, 1914–1918*, vol. 4 (Paris: Masson, 1926–27), p. 205. Hospitals of evacuation were located within the zone controlled by the army but many miles from the front. During the first few months of the war, the French Service de Santé had a policy of sending wounded men directly to the evacuation hospitals after only minimal preliminary treatment. At the hospital, patients would either be treated or sent to the interior. The system had the advantage

of moving casualties away from danger as quickly as possible, but the decided disadvantage of delaying treatment for critical hours. The policy was based on the belief that the war would be short and the theory—soon tragically proved mistaken—that bullet wounds were aseptic. The 1915 introduction of mobile surgical units (*autos-chirurgicals* or *autochirs*) close to the front saved the lives of many men who could not have survived the journey to the evacuation hospitals. See Knibiehler, ed., *Cornettes et blouses blanches,* p. 90; E. Alexander Powell, *Vive la France!* (New York: C. Scribner's Sons, 1915), pp. 224–232.

24. *BP* (April 1908): 43–44.
25. Letter from Minister of War to President of Commission of Budget for War, quoted in *BP* (March 15, 1905): 35–36.
26. Ministry of War, "Notice relative à l'organisation et à l'administration d'un personnel laïque dans les hôpitaux militaires," July 22, 1909, reprinted in *BP* (September 15, 1909): 97–99.
27. *RP,* 22 (January 1908): 373; *BP,* 16 (April 1908): 43–44; Administration générale de l'Assistance Publique à Paris, "Règlement pour le personnel hospitalier," arrêté de 25 mars–19 mai 1910, AAP.
28. Of the ten applicants accepted for admission into the military hospitals, three had trained in Bordeaux—two at the Tondu school and one at the Maison de Santé Protestante. *GM* (June 1908): 87–88; Paul-Louis Lande, "Les Infirmières militaires en France," *GM* (November 1908): 180.
29. Lande, "Les Infirmières militaires en France," pp. 180–181; "Chronique: Les Infirmières militaires," *GM* (December 1908): 209; *GM* (January 1909): 11–12.
30. Circular from Ministry of War to General Command of Army, June 1908, reprinted in *BP,* 16 (September 1908): 103–104; Letter from Médecin Inspecteur Février, Director of Service de Santé of Ministry of War, to Mme. Nathaniel Johnston, Présidente of Sous-Comité du Médoc de la Société de Sécours aux Blessés Militaires, September 28, 1908, reprinted in "Chronique: Une Bonne Leçon," *GM* (April 1909): 65–67; "Au Val-de-Grâce," *GM* (March 1908): 41; *AJN,* 9 (January 1909): 281–82.
31. "Croix-Rouge française," *BP* (September 1908): 102. The Société de Secours aux Blessés Militaires was founded in 1866; the Association des Dames Françaises in 1879; and the Union des Femmes de France, which split off from the ADF, in 1881. An 1892 decree by the Ministry of War during wartime stipulated that the otherwise independent organizations would be administered collectively as the Societies of the French Red Cross. A central committee of the French Red Cross, with representation from all three groups, was created in 1907. John F. Hutchinson, *Champions of Charity: War and the Rise of the Red Cross* (Boulder, Co.: Westview Press, 1996), pp. 256–

268. *RP*, 6 (December 10, 1899): 208–209; *GM* (June 1908): 90. See also Bernard Chevallier, *La Croix-Rouge française: L'Humanitaire tranquille* (Paris: Centurion, 1986); Isabelle Vichniac, *Croix-Rouge: Les Stratèges de la bonne conscience* (Paris: A. Moreau, 1988).

32. "Au Val-de-Grâce," *GM* (March 1908): 41–42; Lande, "Les Infirmières militaires en France," *GM* (November 1908): 189.

33. "Au Val-de-Grâce," *GM* (June 1908): 89.

34. Thébaud, *La Femme au temps de la guerre de 14*, pp. 98–99.

35. Catherine Elston, "L'Hôpital Civil et Militaire d'Elbeuf," *GM* (August 1910): 151.

36. Lavinia L. Dock, "Red Cross of France," *AJN*, 8 (November 1907): 123–124.

37. Félix Régnault, "Les Gardes-malades militaires," *BP* (July 1905): 74–77.

38. Dock, "Red Cross of France," pp. 123–124.

39. Aline Gratuze, *Une Session au Dispensaire-Ecole des Dames Infirmières* (Lyons, 1907); "Rapports du Conseil Supérieur de l'Assistance Publique," CSAP séance du 27 janvier 1921, CSAP fascicule 117, 76–77; *AJN*, 9 (January 1909): 281.

40. Letter from Hamilton to Lavinia L. Dock, April 3, 1910, M. Adelaide Nutting Papers, microfiche 2013.

41. Paul Cornet, "Les Croix-Rouges et les praticiens," *PM* (May 7, 1910): 265.

42. "La Croix Rouge et les sociétés médicales d'arrondissement," *GM* (March 1910): 50.

43. *Le Caducée* (February 19, 1910), quoted in "La Croix Rouge et les sociétés médicales d'arrondissement," p. 52. See also Gilbert, *Les Infirmières en temps de guerre*, p. 15.

44. "La Croix Rouge et les sociétés médicales d'arrondissement," p. 51; Cornet, "Les Croix-Rouges et les praticiens," p. 265.

45. *BP* (April 1908): 43–44.

46. Gratuze, *Une Session au Dispensaire-Ecole*, p. 28.

47. Lande, "Les Infirmières militaires en France," p. 187.

48. Knibiehler, ed., *Cornettes et blouses blanches*, p. 82; Troussaint, *Une Page de l'histoire du Service de Santé Militaire*, p. 133. Many *infirmiers* did not actually tend to the sick and wounded but instead, as *infirmiers d'exploitation*, transported patients and cleaned, or, as *infirmiers commis d'écriture*, held clerical positions. Médecin-inspecteur Heuyer estimated in 1913 that of every 300 *infirmiers*, only 75 actually provided nursing care. Heuyer, *Le Service de Santé, est-il prêt pour la guerre de demain?*, p. 34. A thorough history of the organization of military medicine during the First World War can be found in Mignon, *Le Service de Santé pendant la guerre, 1914–1918*. See also Joseph Toubert, "Historique de l'organisation et du fonctionnement du Service de Santé aux armées pendant la guerre, 1914–1915" (typed mss. in Bibliothèque du Val-de-Grâce), April 15, 1919.

49. Troussaint, *Une Page de l'histoire du Service de Santé*, p. 140.

50. Dorothy Cator, *In a French Military Hospital* (London: Longmans, Green, 1915), p. 25. The American nurse Ellen LaMotte, stationed in a French field hospital just over the border in Belgium, offered a related, though far more sympathetic, account of an *infirmier* who hated the humiliation of his job but continued to perform his duties, knowing that "anything is better than the front line trenches." Ellen N. LaMotte, *The Backwash of War* (New York: G. P. Putnam's Sons, 1934), pp. 48–55. For dissenting views, see E. Tassin, *Cahiers d'une infirmière* (Paris, 1914), p. 16; "French Flag Nursing Corps," *BJN*, 55 (October 2, 1915): 274.

51. Mignon, *Le Service de Santé pendant la guerre*, vol. 1, p. 295.

52. Louis Grandidier, "L'Utilisation des compétences: Ce qu'en dit la Fédération des Services de Santé," *La Bataille syndicaliste*, February 23, 1916. A similar complaint was lodged by Ferdinand Merma in "Le Sursis des infirmiers," *La Bataille syndicaliste*, January 7, 1917.

53. Troussaint, *Une Page de l'histoire du Service de Santé*, pp. 133–134.

54. *Journal officiel*, August 14, 1915, quoted in "French Flag Nursing Corps: Politics and the Wounded," *BJN*, 55 (September 4, 1915): 191.

55. The author did add, generously, that "in spite of these little drawbacks, the French are a charming nation." "Letters from the Front: Nursing French Soldiers," *BJN*, 55 (July 15, 1915): 52.

56. In addition to the regular military hospitals, which were served either by army nurses or by a nursing corps from one of the Red Cross societies, the army also set up *hôpitaux complémentaires*, which were staffed by men and women recruited directly by the Administration Centrale de la Guerre and run by the Service de Santé.

57. During wartime, those medical units—ambulances, dressing stations, train infirmeries, or hospitals—that lay within the *zone d'armée* near the front were controlled by the army general command. Powell, *Vive la France!*, pp. 224–232; Mignon, *Le Service de Santé pendant la guerre*; Léa Bérard, ed., *Au Service de la France: Les Décorées de la Grande Guerre* (s.l.n.d [1919]), p. 1.

58. See, for example, "La Guerre et le travail féminin: La Profession d'infirmière en France," *RP*, 37 (May 15, 1916): 239–240. Léon Abensour, *Les Vaillantes; Héroïnes, martyres et replaçantes* (Paris: Librairie Chapelot, 1917), quoted in Françoise Thébaud, *La Femme au temps de la guerre de 14*, p. 83.

59. "Activité de la Société Française de Secours aux Blessés Militaires pendant la guerre de 1914 à 1918," French Red Cross Library, box 613; Assemblée générale of the Société Française de Secours aux Blessés Militaires (hereafter SSBM), November 23, 1919, French Red Cross library, box 613; "La Croix-Rouge Française: l'Union des Femmes de France et la guerre," September 10, 1915, French Red Cross Library, box 613.

60. Troussaint, *Une Page de l'histoire du Service de Santé*, 142–143; "Expérience d'une apprentie-infirmière," *La Française*, November 15, 1914, p. 2.

61. Statistics on the numbers of degrees issued and numbers of personnel who entered service vary from source to source. One account claimed that the UFF trained over 16,000 nurses and nurses' aides during first year and a half of war. Marie de la Hire, *La Femme française* (Paris: Librairie Jules Tallendier, 1917), p. 72. Another asserted that by December of 1914, the SSBM had issued 12,000 diplomas, the UFF 19,750, and the Association des Dames Françaises (ADF) 6,000. "Miracles de charité: La Croix-Rouge Française," *Lectures pour tous* (January 1915): 629, in French Red Cross Library, box 821. On the requirement for degrees from the various Red Cross societies, see Dr. P. Bouloumié, *Leçons de guerre: La Santé et la guerre* (Paris, 1922), pp. 136–138; "L'Activité de la Société Française de Secours aux Blessés Militaires du 2 août 1914 au 1er 1916," *Bulletin international des sociétés de la Croix-Rouge*, 47 (January 1916), pp. 100–105.

62. Troussaint, *Une Page de l'histoire du Service de Santé*, p. 142.

63. L. Zeys, "Les Femmes et la guerre," *Revue des deux mondes* (September 1, 1916), quoted in Knibiehler, ed., *Cornettes et blouses blanches*, p. 84.

64. "La Croix-Rouge Française: L'Union des Femmes de France et la guerre," September, 10, 1915, in French Red Cross Library, box 613.

65. "Avis aux femmes qui veulent contribuer à la défense de la patrie en danger," *La France de Bordeaux et du Sud-Ouest*, August 2, 1914; "The International Red Cross Society," *BJN*, 55 (August 21, 1915): 154.

66. Troussaint, *Une Page de l'histoire du Service de Santé*, p. 141. On the myth of the World War One nurse, see Thébaud, *La Femme au temps de la guerre de 14*, p. 84. For provocative analyses of gendered definitions of wartime service, see Darrow, "French Volunteer Nursing," and Mary-Louise Roberts, *Civilization without Sexes: Reconstructing Gender in Postwar France, 1917–1927* (Chicago: University of Chicago Press, 1994).

67. Marie de Sardent (Jacques de la Faye), *Feuillets d'epopée. Les Infirmières dans les hôpitaux militaires en temps de guerre* (Auxerre, 1918), p. 20.

68. Mignon, *Le Service de Santé pendant la guerre*, vol. 1, p. 299.

69. Pascal Forthuny, *Le Flambeau* (no date): 397, in French Red Cross Library, box 821.

70. Quoted in "L'Infirmière au chevet du blessé," *BP* (September–October 1914): 101–102.

71. Félix Klein, *The Diary of a French Army Chaplain* (Chicago: A. C. McClurg, 1915), p. 260.

72. Germaine J. Legrix, "Récit d'une infirmière, 27 mai–6 septembre 1918," (typescript, 1966), in French Red Cross Library.

73. "L'Assemblée générale de la Société Française de Secours aux Blessés Militaires, 22 juillet 1917," p. 38, in French Red Cross Library, box 613.

74. Touchet, *Aux Infirmières de France*, p. 74. See also Mignon, *La Service de Santé pendant la guerre*, vol. 1, p. 299.
75. Stephen Liegard, *Le Flambeau* [no date], p. 397, in French Red Cross Library, box 821.
76. Andrée d'Alix, *Le Rôle patriotique des femmes* (Paris: Perrin, 1914), quoted in Hutchinson, *Champions of Charity*, pp. 265–266.
77. L. Sabbatier, "Dans une Gare de rassemblement," *L'Illustration*, 12 (August 1916): 152. For similar allusions in contemporary fiction, see Darrow, "French Volunteer Nursing," pp. 91–92.
78. Jules Combarieu, *Les Jeunes Filles françaises et la guerre* (Paris: Librairie Armand Colin, 1916), p. 136.
79. "La Prière des dames infirmières de France, 1914–1915," in French Red Cross Library, box 821.
80. The doctor also objected to women's presence in military hospitals on the grounds that it was inappropriate for women to come into contact with Germans, Algerians, Senegalese, and other "uncivilized races." Troussaint, *Une Page de l'histoire du Service de Santé*, pp. 140–141. For provacative discussion of the gendered aspects of the mythology of war, see the essays in Miriam Cooke and Angela Woollacott, eds., *Gendering War Talk* (Princeton, N.J.: Princeton University Press, 1993). On women's war journals, see Margaret R. Higonnet, "Not So Quiet in No-Woman's Land," in that volume, pp. 205–226.
81. "Examens de l'Union des Femmes de France," *RP*, 6 (December 10, 1899); Troussaint, *Une Page de l'histoire du Service de Santé*, p. 147.
82. The ADF even issued a *bulletin* to all women who attended two series of eight lessons each. It is unclear whether any institution accepted the document as proof of training. Bouloumié, *Leçons de guerre*, pp. 136–138.
83. Thébaud, *La Femme au temps de la guerre de 14*, p. 85.
84. "The International Red Cross Society," *BJN*, 55 (August 21, 1915): 154. Krafft ran the nursing school La Source in Lausanne, which provided the nursing staff for the Maison de Santé Protestante in Bordeaux before the arrival of Anna Hamilton.
85. As a solution to this problem, Krafft proposed that one of the goals of the next international meeting of the Red Cross societies be "to define the difference of rank between the trained professional nurse and the untrained voluntary helper." "The International Red Cross Society," *BJN*, 55 (August 21, 1915): 154; "Letters from the Front: From Paris," *BJN*, 53 (December 12, 1914): 469.
86. "Les Dames des Croix-Rouges dans les hôpitaux de l'Assistance Publique," *L'Hospitalier* (December 1, 1917); "British Nurses in France," *BJN*, 53 (December 19, 1914), p. 486; "Letters from the Front," *BJN*, 54 (January 16, 1915): 49–50; "Letters from the Front: From Paris," *BJN*, 53 (December 12, 1914): 469.

87. Mabel T. Boardman, *Under the Red Cross Flag* (Philadelphia: J. P. Lippincott, 1915), p. 239.

88. *Le Flambeau* (December 11, 1915): 755.

89. "The International Red Cross Society," p. 154; Letter from Hamilton to Lavinia L. Dock, June 30, 1918, Nutting Collection, microfiche 2013; Letter from Hamilton to M. Adelaide Nutting, January 24, 1920, Nutting Collection, microfiche 2495.

90. "La Guerre et le travail féminin," 239; Dr. P. Tridon, *Qualités et devoirs des infirmières dans les hôpitaux militaires en temps de guerre* (Auxerre, 1918), p. 14.

91. Bérard, ed., *Au Service de la France: Les Décorées de la Grande Guerre* (s.l.n.d [1919]).

92. "Livret de dame infirmière de la Société Française de Secours aux Blessés Militaires," no. 1610, in French Red Cross archive, 221.1.

93. Klein, *The Diary of a French Army Chaplain*, p. 261.

94. Margaret H. Darrow discusses literary and journalistic representations of what she terms the "good" and the "bad" nurse in her "French Volunteer Nursing." For an analysis of contemporary assessments of women's behavior during the war, see Roberts, *Civilization without Sexes*.

95. Sardent, *Feuillets d'epopée*, p. 3; "Letters from the Front," *BJN*, 54 (January 16, 1915), p. 49. By contrast, Anna Hamilton complained that the Red Cross nurses were "much too familiar and flirting with the patients." Letter from Hamilton to M. Adelaide Nutting, January 24, 1920, Nutting Collection, microfiche 2495.

96. Tridon, *Qualités et devoirs des infirmières*, p. 4.

97. "La Croix-Rouge: Mimi Pinson, infirmière," *Le Flambeau* (October 9, 1915): 612.

98. "Miracles de charité: La Croix-Rouge Française," *Lectures pour tous,* 18 (January 1915): 623

99. The Red Cross societies contributed 542,000,000 francs out of a total Service de Santé budget of 2,620,000,000. The SSBM supplied 350,000,000 francs; the UFF, 107,000,000 francs; and the ADF 85,000,000 francs. Toubert, "Historique de l'organisation et du fonctionnement du Service de Santé," p. 133.

100. Mignon, *Le Service de Santé pendant la guerre*, vol. 2, pp. 294–308; Thébaud, *La Femme au temps de la guerre de 14*, pp. 93–94.

101. Klein, *The Diary of a French Army Chaplain*, pp. 241–242.

102. "Letters from the Front: From Paris," *BJN*, 53 (December 12, 1914): 469; "Nursing and the War," *BJN*, 55 (October 23, 1915): 330.

103. Over 127,000 French soldiers suffered from typhoid fever, with a mortality rate of 9.5 percent. By the end of the war, tuberculosis mortality rates had risen to 404 per 100,000 people in the Department of the Seine, compared to

under 200 per 100,000 in New York City and Chicago. The influenza epidemic, meanwhile, struck nearly 195,000 soldiers between April and December of 1918 alone, 12,000 of whom died. Alfred Mignon, who generally had nothing but praise for the Red Cross volunteers, noted that the majority refused to serve in typhoid wards, forcing doctors to draw upon paid nurses. Mignon, *Le Service de Santé pendant la guerre,* vol. 4, pp. 209–210, 705–712, 729; Frank E. Wing, "Fighting Tuberculosis in France," *The Survey,* 42 (May 3, 1919): 178–179.

104. Hamilton to Lavinia L. Dock, April 29, 1917, Nutting Collection, microfiche 2013.

105. Anna Hamilton, "Service des gardes-malades de la Maison de Santé Protestante de Bordeaux pendant la prémière année de guerre," *RP,* 37 (August 15, 1916): 366–368, 372.

106. "A Nursing Pioneer in France," *BJN,* 54 (January 2, 1915): 3; "Nursing and the War: Splendid National Service," *BJN,* 56 (May 6, 1916): 399; Evelyne Diebolt, *La Maison de Santé Protestante de Bordeaux (1863–1934)* (Toulouse: Erès, 1990), p. 95.

107. *BJN,* 53 (December 12, 1914): 466; *BJN,* 53 (December 19, 1914): 487; *BJN,* 57 (November 11, 1916): 388.

108. Thébaud, *La Femme au temps de la guerre de 14,* p. 84; Knibiehler, ed., *Cornettes et blouses blanches,* pp. 82–83; "French Flag Nursing Corps: Politics and the Wounded," *BJN,* 55 (September 4, 1915): 191; "French Flag Nursing Corps," *BJN,* 58 (February 10, 1917): 96.

109. "French Flag Nursing Corps," *BJN,* 54 (March 13, 1915): 213; "British Nurses in France," *BJN,* 53 (December 19, 1914): 486.

110. *BJN,* 55 (July 31, 1915): 93. *BJN,* 54 (May 15, 1915): 414.

111. *BJN,* 54 (January 9, 1915): 28; *BJN,* 58 (January 20, 1917): 41; "Devoted Service Recognized," *BJN,* 61 (November 30, 1918): 334.

112. Letter from Hamilton to Lavinia L. Dock, April 29, 1917, Nutting Collection, microfiche 2013; "Inauguration de l'Hôpital-Ecole Edith-Cavell," *RP,* 37 (November 15, 1916): 550; "Une Institution Féministe: Hôpital-Ecole Edith Cavell," *La Française,* November 11, 1916, p. 2; *Archives de médecine et de pharmacie militaire,* 68 (1917): 804–811; Letter from Hamilton to Lavinia L. Dock, November 28, 1905, Nutting Collection, microfiche 2442; "Un Institut d'infirmières à domiciles," *BP,* 7 (September 15, 1899): 869–870; "Les "Nurses" françaises," *Le Matin,* September 9, 1906; Max Dorville, "A l'Ecole professionnelle d'assistance aux malades," *L'Action,* November 27, 1909.

113. *Archives de médecine et de pharmacie militaire,* 68 (1917): 804; Fernand Laudet, "Le Service de Santé de l'Armée et les services de la Croix-Rouge," *La Revue hebdomadaire* (September 19, 1916); Letter from Hamilton to Lavinia L. Dock, April 29, 1917, Nutting Collection, microfiche 2013.

114. A shortage of personnel also prompted the Ministry of War to allow female

nurses to serve closer to the front from 1915 on. In February 1917, women began replacing male nurses at the front when the latter were drafted into combat troops. By the summer of 1917, a permanent team of eight nurses was attached to every mobile surgical unit. Knibiehler, ed., *Cornettes et blouses blanches*, pp. 89–90; Mignon, *Le Service de Santé pendant la guerre*, vol. 4, p. 205.

115. The temporary nurses drew the same salaries as the regular corps of army nurses instituted in 1908: between 800 and 1354FF annually, plus food, lodging and 100FF for clothing. AD Gironde, 2-R-225; Ministère de la Guerre, Sous-Secrétariat d'Etat du Service de Santé Militaire, circulaire 38 Ci/7, March 8, 1916. See also Knibiehler, ed., *Cornettes et blouses blanches*, pp. 96–98; Bouloumié, *Leçons de guerre*, pp. 142–145.

116. Correspondence between Eudoxie Braud and Prefect of the Gironde, November 1916; January 11, 1917; January 22, 1917; February 19, 1917; April 27, 1917; Correspondence between Marie Louise-Marguérite Vuillet and Prefect of the Gironde, January 6, 1918; Correspondence: Gabrielle Lacaze, Prefect of the Gironde, and Sous-Secrétaire d'Etat du Service de Santé Militaire, March 18, 1917; March 23, 1917; April 4, 1917; June 3, 1917; June 20, 1917; July 7, 1917; December 28, 1917; December 31, 1917; February 23, 1918; June 17, 1918; June 22, 1918, AD, Gironde, 2-R-225; Bouloumié, *Leçons de guerre*, p. 144.

117. François Le Grix, "Le Service de Santé de l'armée et les services de la Croix-Rouge," *La Revue hebdomadaire* (September 19, 1916); "Les Voyages des infirmières," *La Française*, October 4, 1916, p. 2; Bouloumié, *Leçons de guerre*, pp. 143–145.

118. "Décès de M. Louis Renault, président de la Croix-Rouge Française," *Bulletin international de la Croix-Rouge*, 49 (April 1918): 254; "Le Conseil de discipline de la Société Française de Secours," ibid.: 259; Knibiehler, ed., *Cornettes et blouses blanches*, pp. 97–99.

119. Bouloumié, *Leçons de la guerre*, p. 145; Lavinia L. Dock, "Progress in France," *AJN*, 21 (March 1921): 394.

120. Darrow, "French Volunteer Nursing," p. 84.

121. Thébaud, *La Femme au temps de la guerre de 14*, p. 87; Knibiehler, ed., *Cornettes et blouses blanches*, pp. 97–100.

6. Nursing in Postwar France

1. Chaptal, a prime mover in the establishment of the first tuberculosis dispensary in Paris, also directed the Oeuvre des Tuberculeux Adultes, and served as president of the Commission de l'Enfance de l'Office d'Hygiène Sociale de la Seine. Among Chaptal's numerous other initiatives, she opened a well-baby

clinic in 1901 and helped build housing for the poor that included a cooperative shop where the sale of alcohol was strictly forbidden. Chaptal was one of six female members of the CSAP, which, in 1921, included 130 politicians, medical professionals, hospital administrators, members of the clergy, and representatives of philanthropic organizations. "Annexe I: Composition du Conseil Supérieur de l'Assistance Publique," January 26, 1921, CSAP fascicule 117, pp. 130–134. For detailed descriptions of Chaptal's career, see Yvonne Knibiehler, ed., *Cornettes et blouses blanches: Les Infirmières dans la société française, 1880–1980* (Paris: Hachette, 1984), pp. 109–112; "Mlle. Chaptal," *South African Nursing Record* (September 1930): 315–316.

2. "Rapports du Conseil Supérieur de l'Assistance Publique," (hereafter CSAP report), January 27, 1921, fascicule 117, p. 68.

3. CSAP report, January 27, 1921, fascicule 117, p. 100.

4. Ibid., pp. 100–101.

5. Ibid., p. 69.

6. Mme. Pigeon-Gillot, "Examen d'Etat," *BP,* 16 (September 1908): 97–98.

7. *Fédération des Services de Santé de France et des Colonies, IIe Congrès corporatif, Lyon, 1908* (Bourges: Imprimerie ouvrier du centre ouvriers, syndiqués, et fédérés, 1908), pp. 29–32.

8. *Fédération des Services de Santé de France et des Colonies, Ve Congrès corporatif, Paris, 1912* (Bourges: Imprimerie ouvrier du centre ouvriers, syndiqués, et fédérés, 1912), p. 151.

9. "Contre la réintégration des soeurs dans les hôpitaux," *L'Humanité,* November 11, 1913.

10. *Le Petit Méridional,* December 23, 1913, quoted in *L'Ouvrier sanitaire* (s.d.) in AN F[7] 13814.

11. CSAP report, January 27, 1921, fascicule 117, p. 85. Dron, who also served intermittently as mayor of Tourcoing between 1889 and 1930, was a staunch promoter of public hygiene and was well known among his constituents as "the doctor of . . . the disinherited." He devoted much of his energy to the improvement of health care for working-class infants, children, and new mothers. Mary Lynn Stewart, *Women, Work, and the French State: Labour Protection and Social Patriarchy, 1879–1919* (Kingston, Ontario: McGill-Queen's University Press, 1989), pp. 34–35.

12. Paul Strauss, "Bulletin," *RP,* 42 (February 15, 1921): 99; "Les Mécontentes," *La Française,* March 29, 1919. *RP,* 40 (June 15, 1919): 344.

13. *Procès-verbaux* of the CSAP, November 19, 1920; Police report of meeting of Syndicat du Personnel Non-Gradé, December 11, 1919, AN F[7]13814.

14. CSAP report, January 27, 1921, fascicule 117, p. 77. Ironically, one of the earliest advocates of state regulation of the nursing profession and of a state nursing diploma was Dr. Bouloumié, Secretary General of the Union des

Femmes de France, one of the three French Red Cross relief organizations. "Illégalité et Légalité," *BP,* 19 (August 15, 1911).

15. Letter from Hamilton to Miss Maxwell, September 24, 1919, Nutting Collection, microfiche 2495.

16. CSAP report, January 27, 1921, fascicule 117, p. 83.

17. AAP, *Procès-verbaux* of the CSAP, June 5, 1919; June 26, 1919.

18. In opposing the eight-hour work day, many doctors and hospital administrators argued that hospital work should not be considered the equivalent of factory work and that nurses and other personnel should not be forced to interrupt their service because of artificial work rules. Administrators and politicians were also concerned about the cost of hiring a third shift of workers. AAP, *Procès-verbaux* of the CSAP, June 5, 1919. On the campaign for and application of the Eight-Hour Day in general, see Gary Cross, *A Quest for Time: The Reduction of Work in Britain and France, 1840–1940* (Berkeley: University of California Press, 1989), esp. pp. 129–149.

19. CSAP report, January 27, 1921, fascicule 117, p. 84; Letters from Anna Hamilton to M. Adelaide Nutting, January 19, 1921; July 10, 1920, Nutting Collection, microfiche 2495.

20. Judith G. Coffin explores the nineteenth century roots of this mistrust, in Coffin, *The Politics of Women's Work: The Paris Garment Trades, 1750-1915* (Princeton, N.J.: Princeton University Press, 1996); "Social Science Meets Sweated Labor: Reinterpreting Women's Work in Late Nineteenth-Century France," *Journal of Modern History,* 63 (June 1991): 230–270; and "Credit, Consumption, and Images of Women's Desires: Selling the Sewing Machine in Late Nineteenth Century France," *French Historical Studies,* 18 (Spring 1994): 749–783. For a discussion of the impact of the war on perceptions of women's work from the perspective of state policy, see Susan Pedersen, *Family, Dependence, and the Origins of the Welfare State: Britain and France, 1914–1945* (Cambridge: Cambridge University Press, 1993), pp. 79–133.

21. On the gendered implications of social retrenchment in the post-war period, see Mary Louise Roberts, *Civilization without Sexes: Reconstructing Gender in Postwar France, 1917–1927* (Chicago: University of Chicago Press, 1994).

22. B. R. Mitchell, *European Historical Statistics, 1750–1970,* (New York, 1978), quoted in Karen Offen, "Depopulation, Nationalism, and Feminism in Fin-de-Siècle France," *American Historical Review,* 89 (June 1984): 650–52; Pedersen, *Family, Dependence, and the Origins of the Welfare State,* p. 60.

23. Alcoholism and venereal disease were also identified as "plagues" during the postwar period, but the campaigns against them relied less heavily on the efforts of nurses.

24. Alisa Klaus, "Depopulation and Race Suicide: Maternalism and Pronatalist Ideologies in France and the United States," in Seth Koven and Sonya Michel,

eds., *Mothers of a New World: Maternalist Politics and the Origins of Welfare States* (New York: Routledge, 1993), pp. 188–212; see also Alisa Klaus, *Every Child a Lion: The Origins of Maternal and Infant Health Policy in the United States and France, 1890–1920* (Ithaca, N.Y.: Cornell University Press, 1993). On the impact of concerns about women's (especially mothers') health on labor legislation and on the political debates surrounding the passage of the Strauss Law, see Stewart, *Women, Work, and the French State,* pp. 149–190.

25. Jacques Léonard, *La Médecine entre les pouvoirs et les savoirs* (Paris: Aubier, 1981), p. 317.

26. "L'Assemblée générale de l'Union des Femmes de France en juillet 1916," *Bulletin international des Sociétés de la Croix-Rouge,* 48 (January 1917): 92; "L'Assemblée générale de la Croix-Rouge française en juillet 1918," *Bulletin international des Sociétés de la Croix-Rouge,* 49 (October 1918): 515–516; Foster Rhea Dulles, *The American Red Cross: A History* (New York: Harper, 1950), pp. 176–177, 195–199; Lion Murard and Patrick Zylberman, "La Mission Rockefeller en France et la création du Comité National de Défense contre la Tuberculose," *Revue d'histoire moderne et contemporaine,* 34 (April-June 1987): 267–273; Klaus, "Depopulation and Race Suicide," pp. 197–198.

27. Léonie Chaptal, "La rôle de la femme dans la prophylaxie antituberculose," *BP,* 20 (July 1912): 73–74. The visiting nurse had already made her debut in France: in 1908 Hamilton's Maison de Santé Protestante inaugurated a program for "Gardes-malades visiteuses des pauvres." The role of the *garde-malade visiteuse* was strictly limited to the observation and evaluation of the health and living conditions of the poor. In cases where inhabitants required medical care, she was to direct them to the nearest dispensary or encourage them to call on the local doctor supplied by the *bureau de bienfaisance* (welfare office). Anna Hamilton, "La Garde-malade visiteuse des pauvres," *GM* (May 1909): 73–80; (August 1910): 158–161.

28. *Actes du cinquième Congrès National d'Assistance Publique et de Bienfaisance Privée, troisième question: L'Infirmière dans l'assistance à domicile* (Nantes: Imprimerie de A. Dugas, 1911); Dr. Gustave Drouineau, "L'Infirmière dans l'assistance à domicile," *RP,* 29 (October 15, 1911): 634–658; Anna Hamilton, "La Garde-malade visiteuse des pauvres au Congrès de Nantes," *GM* (October 1911): 173–179.

29. "Les Infirmières-visiteuses de France et la lutte anti-tuberculeuse," *La Française,* February 3, 1917; "Carrières féminines," *La Française,* December 23, 1916.

30. "L'Association des Infirmières-visiteuses de France," *BP,* 22 (April 15, 1914): 38.

31. Annual salaries were a comparatively high 2,200 frances for those working

in hospitals, dispensaries, and homes, and ranged from 1,000 to 1,500 francs for nurses working in the sanitary stations, where they also received food, clothing, and lodging. "Infirmières visiteuses," *La Française,* May 2, 1914; "Carrières féminines," *La Française,* December 23, 1916; "Les Infirmières visiteuses de France et la lutte antituberculeuse," *La Française,* February 3, 1917.

32. Quoted in Knibiehler, ed., *Cornettes et blouses blanches,* p. 143.

33. Cliffort G. Grulee, "The Work of the Children's Bureau of the American Red Cross in Lyons," *American Journal of Diseases of Children,* 16 (October 1918): 220–225. As Mary Louise Roberts points out, *puériculture* was based on the belief "that women needed detailed instruction and constant medical surveillance in order to raise their children correctly." Roberts, *Civilization without Sexes,* pp. 207, 127–128, fn.328. See also, Yvonne Knibiehler and Catherine Fouquet, *La Femme et les médecins: Analyse historique* (Paris: Hachette, 1983).

34. Clara D. Noyes, "Le 'Nursing' en Europe," *Revue internationale de la Croix Rouge,* 3 (May 15, 1921): 448; *Proceedings of the Medical Conference held at the Invitation of the Committee of Red Cross Societies* (Geneva: Atar S.A., 1919), p. 135.

35. Adolphe d'Espine, "Puériculture et Croix-Rouge," p. 939; "Revue des Congrès," *Annales d'hygiène publique et de médecine légale,* 32 (July 1919): 50–57.

36. Knibiehler, ed., *Cornettes et blouses blanches,* pp. 144–145; Henry P. Davison, "The American Red Cross in the Great War, 1917–1919," in Donald S. Howard, ed., *Administration of Relief Abroad* (New York: Russel Sage Foundation, 1943), p. 12; William Palmer Lucas, "For the Children of France," *The Red Cross Magazine,* 13 (August 1918): 62–68; CSAP report, January 27, 1921, fascicule 117, p. 87

37. CSAP report, January 27, 1921, fascicule 117, pp. 85–86.

38. "L'Union des oeuvres charitables," *Revue internationale de la Croix-Rouge,* 1 (October 15, 1919): 1205.

39. Thérèse Casevitz, "Les Infirmières d'hygiène," *La Française,* May 15, 1920.

40. Ibid., June 19, 1920; July 24, 1920.

41. They also treated minor injuries and illnesses and monitored potential transmitters of contagious diseases.

42. CSAP report, January 27, 1921; Letter from Hamilton to Miss Maxwell, September 24, 1919, Nutting Collection, microfiche 2495; M. Letellier, "Les Questions d'enseignement professionnel à la Réunion de Paris du Conseil Européen pour la formation des infirmières," *L'Infirmière française* (1923): 27–28.

43. Evelyne Diebolt, *La Maison de Santé Protestante de Bordeaux (1863–1934)* (Toulouse: Erès, 1990), pp. 118–120.

44. Hamilton approved of the decree in general, but deplored the fact that Léonie Chaptal, her long-standing professional rival, had played such a dominant role in its formulation. Hamilton's correspondence with nursing leaders in the United States reveals an intense resentment toward Chaptal and her fellow "lady-reformers" in Paris, who "received far more official attention than they deserved simply because they lived in the capital city . . ." Letter from Hamilton to Lavinia L. Dock, August 21, 1924, Nutting Collection, microfiche 2496.

45. "Arrêté ministériel nommant les membres du Conseil de Perfectionnement des Ecoles d'Infirmières," *RP*, 43 (October 15, 1922): 501–502.

Index